CORTISOL

DETOX

DIET-PLAN

A Proven Method to Burn Fat Fast, Lose Weight Naturally, and Restore Hormonal Balance

DEBORAH DONALD

COPYRIGHT

© 2025 **Deborah Donald**
All rights reserved.

This publication is designed to provide accurate and authoritative information regarding the subject matter covered. It is sold with the understanding that the author and publisher are not engaged in rendering medical, health, or any other kind of personal professional services. If medical or other expert assistance is required, the services of a competent professional should be sought.

First edition published in 2025 by Avalon Publishing House
Printed in the United States of America.

Dedication

To everyone who has ever felt overwhelmed by the weight of stress and its impact on your health—this book is for you.

To the warriors who strive for balance, the seekers of wellness, and the believers in lasting change.

And to the ones who remind us daily that health is a gift worth fighting for—thank you for inspiring this journey.

Acknowledgments

No book is created in isolation, and this one is no exception. It takes a village of support, wisdom, and encouragement to bring an idea to life.

First, my heartfelt gratitude to the scientists, nutritionists, and wellness experts who continue to explore and share their insights into the complex world of hormones, stress, and health. Your dedication inspires me daily.

To my family and friends, thank you for standing by me, cheering me on, and reminding me why this work matters. Your patience during the long writing hours and your belief in me have been my anchor.

To my readers—past, present, and future—thank you for trusting me to be a part of your wellness journey. Your stories of resilience and success fuel my passion to keep learning and sharing.

Finally, to the quiet moments of struggle and reflection that became the foundation for this book—thank you for teaching me that balance is always worth pursuing.

This book is the culmination of countless hours of learning, experimenting, and growing. It is my hope that it brings you clarity, peace, and a renewed sense of vitality. Thank you for letting me be part of your path to a healthier, happier life.

Contents

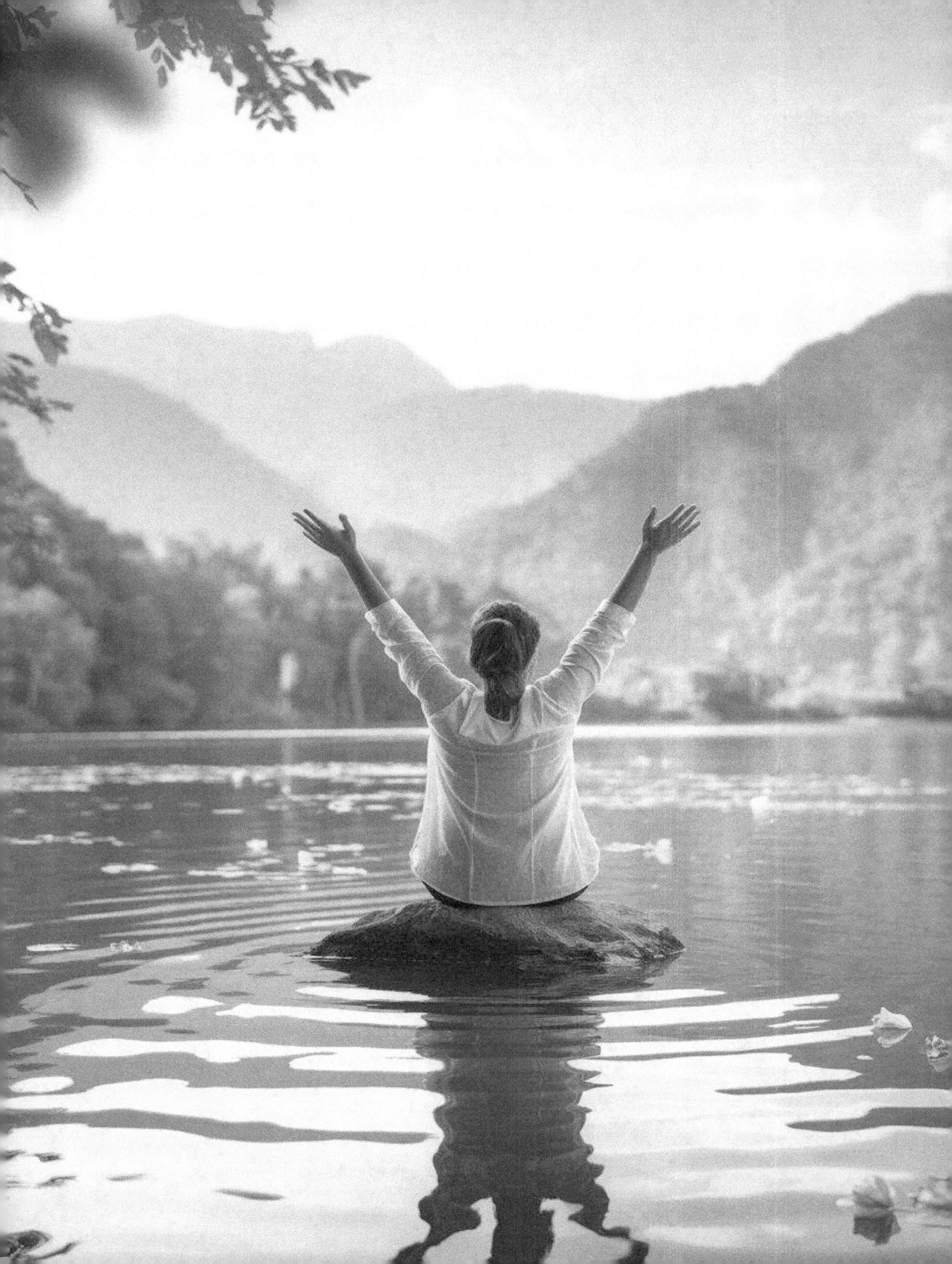

Preface

Stress has become the silent shadow in our modern lives, weaving its way into our routines, our relationships, and even our health. I've felt its grip, just as many of you have. For years, I struggled to understand why no amount of effort seemed to bring the calm and clarity I desperately sought. Then, I discovered the profound connection between cortisol, the body's stress hormone, and the many ways it influences everything—from energy and weight to mood and overall well-being.

This book isn't just about information; it's about transformation. My goal is to guide you through understanding the why behind your body's signals and offer actionable, simple steps to reclaim your balance. You'll find practical tools, science-backed advice, and recipes that nurture your body and soul.

The journey outlined here is not about perfection—it's about progress. Whether you're just starting to address stress's impact on your health or looking for ways to refine your wellness routine, this book is your companion, filled with encouragement and expertise to keep you moving forward.

So, take a deep breath, turn the page, and let's explore how to live a life that's lighter, healthier, and truly yours.

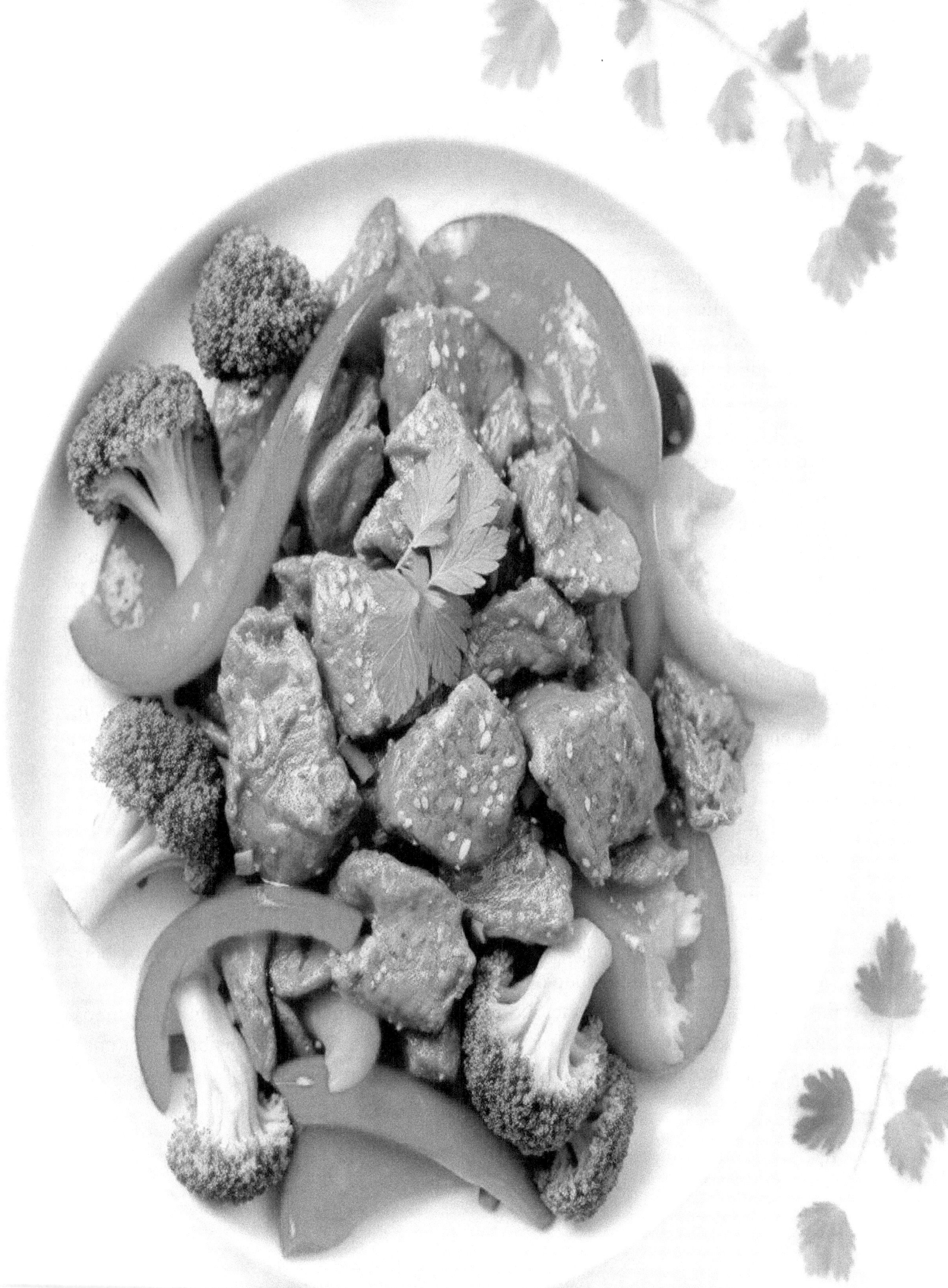

Introduction: Your Hormonal Reset Begins Here

Let me take you back to a moment that changed everything for me. It was a regular Tuesday afternoon. I was sitting in my doctor's office, trying to explain why I felt like a stranger in my own body. I was constantly tired but couldn't sleep, my jeans didn't fit anymore despite eating "right," and I had this nagging feeling that something wasn't quite right. My doctor looked over my lab results and uttered a word that, at the time, didn't mean much to me: cortisol.

Like many people, I had no idea how much power this single hormone had over my health. All I knew was that stress was part of life. Work stress, family stress, money stress—it's just how the world works, **right?** What I didn't realize was that this "normal" stress was wreaking havoc on my body. My weight, energy, and mood weren't random. They were signals that my cortisol levels were out of balance.

As I dug deeper, I learned that I wasn't alone. Millions of people feel overwhelmed, burned out, and disconnected from their bodies. That's why this book exists: to help you understand how cortisol could be the key to unlocking your energy, metabolism, and overall well-being. This isn't just a diet plan—it's a complete reset for your health.

Why Cortisol Matters in Today's World

Stress isn't what it used to be. Thousands of years ago, our stress response was designed to help us survive immediate threats. Imagine you're a hunter-gatherer, and a lion leaps out from the bushes. Your body floods with cortisol to sharpen your senses, give you a burst of energy, and focus all your resources on getting away safely. Once the danger passed, cortisol levels would drop, and your body would return to its natural state of balance.

Fast forward to today, and the "lion" isn't a wild animal—it's your email inbox, financial worries, traffic jams, or trying to juggle a million responsibilities at once. Unlike our ancestors, we rarely get the chance to recover fully. Our bodies stay stuck in "fight or flight" mode, producing cortisol at levels that throw everything out of sync.

Here's why that's a problem:

- **Weight Gain**: Cortisol triggers cravings for sugary, high-fat foods, which were once vital for survival but now lead to stubborn belly fat.
- **Poor Sleep**: Elevated cortisol keeps your mind racing at night, disrupting the deep, restorative sleep your body needs.
- **Low Energy**: Chronic stress depletes your energy reserves, leaving you feeling tired no matter how much rest you get.
- **Mood Swings**: Imbalanced cortisol affects your brain's chemistry, making you feel anxious, irritable, or even depressed.

The goal of this book is to break that cycle. By understanding cortisol and taking practical steps to rebalance it, you can restore your health, shed unwanted weight, and regain the calm energy you need to thrive.

Let's address a common misconception: stress isn't the enemy. It's a natural part of life, and in small doses, it can even be motivating. The problem arises when stress becomes chronic and cortisol levels remain elevated. The good news? You don't need extreme diets, expensive supplements, or grueling workouts to fix this.

This book is built on simple, science-backed solutions:

- **Balanced Nutrition**: The foods you eat can either fuel your stress or help your body relax. We'll focus on whole, nourishing ingredients that stabilize blood sugar and support healthy cortisol levels.
- **Lifestyle Changes**: Small shifts in your daily routine—like prioritizing sleep or adding mindfulness practices—can make a big difference.
- **A Manageable Plan**: This isn't about perfection. It's about progress. You'll find realistic strategies that fit into your life, not the other way around.

Whether you're here to lose weight, boost your energy, or simply feel better in your own skin, this journey is about more than quick fixes. It's about building habits that last.

Many of us think of stress as purely mental—a state of mind we just have to "push through." But stress has very real, physical effects on your body, and ignoring it won't make those effects disappear. Here are some common myths you might believe about stress, weight, or hormones:

- **"I'm just getting older."**
  While it's true that metabolism changes with age, much of what we attribute to aging—like weight gain, fatigue, or brain fog—can actually be linked to cortisol imbalances.
- **"If I eat less and exercise more, I'll lose weight."**
  Over-exercising or severely restricting calories can backfire, increasing cortisol levels and making weight loss even harder.
- **"Stress is just part of life."**
  While we can't eliminate stress entirely, we can change how our bodies respond to it. The goal isn't to avoid stress but to build resilience.

Understanding these truths is the first step toward making meaningful changes.

Let me tell you about Sarah, a client who came to me desperate for a solution. She was a busy mom with a demanding job, and she felt like she was constantly running on empty. No matter how hard she worked out or how "clean" her diet was, the scale wouldn't budge, and her energy levels were at an all-time low.

When we looked at her lifestyle, the culprit became clear: chronic stress. Sarah was skipping meals, sleeping only five hours a night, and pushing herself to the limit with intense workouts. Her cortisol levels were through the roof.

Together, we made small but impactful changes. We adjusted her diet to include more calming, nutrient-dense foods. She swapped high-intensity exercise for yoga and walking. Most importantly, she started prioritizing sleep and self-care. Within weeks, Sarah noticed a difference. She had more energy, her mood improved, and the weight she'd been struggling with started to come off naturally.

Sarah's story isn't unique. It's proof that when you give your body the tools it needs to thrive, it responds.

This book is your guide to a healthier, more balanced life. Whether you're feeling overwhelmed, struggling with your weight, or just looking for a way to feel more like yourself again, the solutions are within reach.

Together, we'll explore how to reset your cortisol levels using practical strategies and nourishing recipes. You'll learn how to listen to your body, manage stress more effectively, and create a lifestyle that supports your goals.

The journey won't be about perfection—it'll be about learning, growing, and finding what works for you. So take a deep breath. You're in the right place, and the best is yet to come.

Part 1: Understanding Cortisol – The Stress Hormone Unmasked

CHAPTER 1

WHAT IS CORTISOL, AND WHY DOES IT MATTER?

Cortisol is one of those things you may have heard about, but never fully understood. It's often associated with stress, but its role goes far beyond just dealing with pressure. Think of cortisol as your body's built-in alarm system, always on standby to help you handle life's challenges. But what happens when this system gets out of sync? That's where the problems begin. Let's break down cortisol, why it's crucial for your well-being, and how it affects everything from your energy to your mood.

The Cortisol Curve: Your Body's Natural Rhythm
Imagine your day as a rollercoaster, and cortisol is the seatbelt that keeps you in place. Normally, cortisol follows a daily rhythm, often referred to as the "cortisol curve." In the morning, when your body needs to wake up, cortisol levels rise. This surge helps you feel alert and energized, preparing you to take on the day. By evening, cortisol levels naturally decrease, allowing you to wind down and sleep.

For most people, this rhythm works without them thinking about it—until it doesn't. Stress, poor sleep, and unhealthy habits can disrupt the cortisol curve, leading to imbalances that affect your body in many ways. When cortisol stays high for too long—thanks to constant stress, late nights, or poor diet—it can turn from a helpful ally into a major source of imbalance.

Cortisol and Energy: The Constant Tug-of-War
Now, let's talk about how cortisol affects your energy. Normally, when cortisol is balanced, it helps your body respond to stress and gives you a healthy burst of energy when you need it most. Picture it like a cup of coffee in your system—just enough to keep you alert but not too much to leave you jittery.

But here's the kicker: if your cortisol levels are consistently elevated, your energy can suffer. This is especially true when cortisol is high at night, tricking your body into thinking it's still "go-time." You might find yourself lying awake at 2 a.m., mind racing with thoughts, unable to fall asleep because your cortisol is still on high alert.

Real-life example: Take Sarah, a mother of two with a full-time job. Every day, she faces constant demands at work, keeps her kids busy, and somehow tries to manage a household. Sarah's cortisol is constantly elevated because she's always on the go, running on fumes but never getting enough downtime. As a result, she feels wired at night, has trouble falling asleep, and wakes up exhausted. Cortisol has her trapped in a cycle of chronic fatigue.

When cortisol is out of whack like this, you feel drained, unmotivated, and it's tough to find that energy to do the things you enjoy.

Cortisol and Weight: The Hidden Connection

Cortisol is also a major player when it comes to your weight. When cortisol levels are consistently high, your body thinks it's in a state of emergency. And what does the body do in an emergency? It stores fat. More specifically, cortisol encourages your body to store fat around your abdomen—one of the most stubborn areas to lose weight.

Here's why: cortisol triggers the release of insulin, a hormone that helps control blood sugar levels. When cortisol is chronically elevated, your blood sugar stays high for longer periods, prompting your body to store excess sugar as fat. It's like your body is preparing for a famine that never comes.

Let's take another real-life example: Tim, a guy in his late 30s, always had a lean build in his younger years. But after years of working long hours at a stressful job, he noticed his waistline expanding, even though his diet hadn't changed much. Tim's cortisol was elevated due to the constant pressure at work, and his body was holding on to that belly fat. No matter how many crunches he did, that stubborn fat wouldn't budge.

So, if you're finding it harder to shed pounds despite eating right and exercising, it's not just about what you eat or how much you move. Cortisol could be working against you, storing fat when it should be burning it.

Cortisol and Sleep: The Disrupted Cycle

Sleep is another area where cortisol plays a pivotal role. The relationship between cortisol and sleep is like a balancing act. When cortisol levels are too high at night, it's nearly impossible to relax and fall asleep. That's why many people who are stressed out report tossing and turning at night—cortisol is keeping their bodies in a state of heightened alertness.

Now, think about when you're feeling relaxed—cortisol drops, and another hormone, melatonin, takes over to help you sleep. But when cortisol doesn't drop the way it's supposed to, it prevents your body from making that natural transition into sleep mode. The result? A restless night, waking up tired, and starting the cycle all over again.

Real-life example: Rachel has always been a night owl, but after having children, she found herself staying up late to catch some quiet time after a busy day. Her mind was always racing, and she couldn't wind down. The high cortisol levels at night left her feeling restless and tired, no matter how many hours she spent in bed. Over time, Rachel's body started to feel worn down, her mood worsened, and the weight slowly crept on.

Sleep and cortisol go hand in hand. When cortisol is balanced, sleep comes easily. But when it's out of sync, sleep quality suffers, making you more tired, more stressed, and less able to focus during the day.

Cortisol and Emotions: The Mood Rollercoaster

You've probably noticed that when you're under stress, your mood takes a hit. That's because cortisol has a direct impact on your brain and emotions. When cortisol levels are elevated, it can contribute to feelings of anxiety, irritability, and even depression. It changes the balance of neurotransmitters in your brain, leading to mood swings and emotional instability.

Real-life example: John was dealing with some tough personal situations and noticed he was becoming more short-tempered. Small issues that never bothered him before suddenly felt overwhelming. His energy was low, and he felt disconnected from his friends and family. This emotional rollercoaster was a direct result of his cortisol imbalance. His body was stuck in a chronic stress mode, and his mental health was suffering as a result.

Cortisol's effect on mood is real and often overlooked. When it's imbalanced, it can make everything feel harder—whether it's managing relationships, work, or just getting through the day. Finding ways to reduce stress and rebalance cortisol can make a huge difference in how you feel emotionally.

Bringing It All Together

So, why does cortisol matter? Because it's deeply connected to your energy, weight, sleep, and mood. When your cortisol levels are balanced, everything works the way it should. You feel energized, you sleep better, your metabolism functions properly, and your mood remains stable.

But when cortisol is out of balance, it can disrupt your body's natural rhythms, leading to fatigue, weight gain, poor sleep, and emotional struggles. Understanding this connection is the first step toward reclaiming your health and well-being.

As you move forward in this book, you'll learn how to reset your cortisol, reduce stress, and restore balance. It's not about being perfect—it's about making small, manageable changes that allow your body to return to its natural rhythm.

Are you ready to get started? Your journey toward a balanced, energized, and healthier life begins now.

CHAPTER 2

THE SILENT SABOTEUR: HIDDEN TRIGGERS OF HIGH CORTISOL

Cortisol is often called the "stress hormone," but it doesn't always need a major crisis to get activated. Many of us live in a state of static stress, where everyday habits, environmental factors, and even the foods we eat keep cortisol levels elevated without us even realizing it. These triggers are sneaky, building up over time until the effects are impossible to ignore.

In this chapter, we'll uncover some of the most common hidden triggers that push cortisol into overdrive, how they affect your body, and how to spot them in your own life.

Everyday Triggers That Raise Cortisol

1. Poor Diet: What You Eat (or Don't Eat) Matters

Your diet is one of the biggest factors influencing cortisol. When your body lacks proper nutrients or is overloaded with unhealthy foods, it can trigger stress responses that keep cortisol levels high.

- **Sugar and Processed Foods**: Ever feel that crash after eating a sugary snack? High-sugar diets cause blood sugar spikes, followed by sharp drops, putting stress on your body. Your adrenal glands release more cortisol to stabilize blood sugar levels, leading to a vicious cycle.
- **Caffeine Overload**: While a cup of coffee can give you a temporary boost, too much caffeine stimulates cortisol production, especially when paired with insufficient sleep or stress.
- **Skipping Meals**: Skipping meals—or going long stretches without eating— forces your body into "survival mode." This signals cortisol to rise, as your body believes it needs to conserve energy.

- **Low Nutrient Intake**: Diets low in vitamins, minerals, and healthy fats deprive your body of the building blocks it needs to function, indirectly raising cortisol as your body works harder to compensate.

Tip: To avoid cortisol spikes, aim for balanced meals with protein, healthy fats, and complex carbohydrates. Whole foods like leafy greens, nuts, seeds, and lean proteins help maintain steady energy and reduce stress on your body.

2. Chronic Stress: The Pressure Cooker Effect

Stress doesn't just come from deadlines or arguments—it can also stem from mental overload, constant multitasking, or even unspoken worries. While stress itself isn't inherently bad (it can motivate us to act), prolonged stress keeps your cortisol stuck in the "on" position.

- **Emotional Stress**: Unresolved conflicts, financial worries, or feelings of overwhelm keep your adrenal glands working overtime, pumping out cortisol even when the situation doesn't require it.
- **Workload and Time Pressure**: Many people underestimate how much their packed schedules affect their health. Working long hours without breaks can lead to adrenal fatigue and burnout.
- **Environmental Stress**: Constant noise, cluttered spaces, or even exposure to harmful toxins in cleaning products and plastics can subtly increase cortisol levels over time.

Tip: Begin identifying what stresses you most by keeping a stress journal for a week. Write down what situations or tasks feel overwhelming and how you physically react (e.g., racing heart, tight chest). Awareness is the first step to managing triggers.

3. Sleep Deprivation: The Silent Cortisol Booster

Sleep is when your body restores itself, balancing hormones and repairing stress-related damage. Without enough quality sleep, your cortisol levels remain elevated longer than they should.

- **Late Nights**: Staying up late—whether working, scrolling on your phone, or binging your favorite show—disrupts the natural cortisol rhythm. Ideally, cortisol should be at its lowest when you're winding down for bed.
- **Interrupted Sleep**: Waking up frequently during the night interrupts the deep restorative phases of sleep, leaving your body in a state of static alertness.
- **Inconsistent Sleep Schedules**: Irregular sleep patterns (like sleeping in on weekends and waking early on weekdays) confuse your internal clock, leading to poor cortisol regulation.

Tip: Aim for consistent bedtimes, limit screen time before sleep, and create a calming pre-sleep routine, such as reading or practicing deep breathing. Small changes can lead to big improvements in how your body manages cortisol.

4. Hormonal Imbalances: When Stress Hijacks Your System

Prolonged stress doesn't just affect cortisol—it also disrupts other hormones that are interconnected with it.

- **Insulin**: Chronic stress leads to insulin resistance, where your cells stop responding to insulin as effectively. This results in higher blood sugar levels and a greater demand for cortisol to keep things stable.
- **Thyroid Hormones**: Stress can suppress thyroid hormone production, slowing your metabolism and leaving you feeling fatigued.
- **Sex Hormones**: Elevated cortisol diverts resources away from the production of reproductive hormones like estrogen and testosterone. This can lead to issues like irregular cycles, low libido, or mood swings.

Tip: If you suspect hormonal imbalances, talk to a healthcare professional who can recommend tests to assess your cortisol levels and other key hormones.

How to Identify Your Cortisol Triggers

Understanding what's causing your high cortisol is the first step to regaining balance. Use the checklist below to evaluate potential triggers in your own life.

Cortisol Trigger Checklist

Tick off any of the following that apply to you:
1. **Dietary Habits**
    - Do you consume sugary snacks or drinks daily?
    - Do you skip meals or go long hours without eating?
    - Is caffeine a regular part of your day, especially in the afternoon or evening?
2. **Stress Levels**
    - Do you feel overwhelmed by work, family, or financial responsibilities?
    - Do you often feel irritable, anxious, or emotionally drained?
    - Is your schedule packed with little time for breaks?
3. **Sleep Patterns**
    - Do you get less than 6–7 hours of sleep most nights?
    - Do you wake up feeling tired, even after a full night's rest?
    - Are your sleep and wake times inconsistent?
4. **Lifestyle and Environment**
    - Are you exposed to loud noises, bright screens, or cluttered environments daily?
    - Do you rely on convenience foods or takeout more than home-cooked meals?
    - Do you lack time for self-care or relaxation?
5. **Physical Symptoms**
    - Have you noticed stubborn weight gain, especially around your midsection?
    - Do you frequently feel fatigued, even without a clear reason?
    - Are you experiencing mood swings or a lower tolerance for stress?

If you answered "yes" to several questions, it's likely that cortisol triggers are playing a significant role in your health. But don't worry—recognizing the problem is a powerful step toward finding solutions.

Taking Back Control

Cortisol may be the silent saboteur, but the good news is that it's also responsive to positive changes. By adjusting your diet, managing stress, prioritizing sleep, and addressing hormonal imbalances, you can reset your cortisol levels and start feeling better.

In the next chapter, we'll explore specific foods and nutrients that help regulate cortisol, so you can take charge of your health and create a lifestyle that supports balance and well-being. The power to overcome these triggers is in your hands, and this book is here to guide you every step of the way.

CHAPTER 3

THE COST OF IMBALANCE

In today's fast-paced world, stress is almost like a badge of honor. But living with chronic stress has a hidden price, one that your body pays over time. Elevated cortisol levels might feel manageable in the short term, but the long-term consequences are far from static. From subtle warning signs to life-altering health conditions, an unchecked cortisol imbalance can wreak havoc on your physical and emotional well-being.

Let's uncover the ripple effects of chronically elevated cortisol, so you can understand why resetting your levels is essential to restoring your health and vitality.

The Long-Term Toll of Elevated Cortisol

When cortisol stays high, your body operates in a constant state of "fight or flight." While this response is helpful in emergencies, it's not designed to be permanent. Chronic elevation disrupts the natural rhythm of your body, leading to a cascade of negative effects.

1. Weight Gain and Fat Storage

Cortisol has a direct impact on how your body stores and uses energy. High levels signal your body to store fat, especially around your midsection. This isn't just about aesthetics—abdominal fat is linked to higher risks of cardiovascular disease and diabetes.

- **Why It Happens**: Elevated cortisol increases appetite and cravings for high-calorie, sugary foods. It also promotes fat storage as a protective mechanism, preparing your body for the perceived stress.

- **The Numbers Speak**: Studies show that individuals with high cortisol levels are 2.5 times more likely to develop obesity, particularly central obesity.

2. Metabolic Syndrome: A Cluster of Risks

Metabolic syndrome isn't a single condition but a group of risk factors that often travel together: high blood pressure, high blood sugar, abnormal cholesterol levels, and excess abdominal fat. Elevated cortisol can directly contribute to each of these.

- **Insulin Resistance**: Cortisol interferes with insulin, making it harder for your body to regulate blood sugar. This can eventually lead to type 2 diabetes.
- **Hypertension**: Chronic stress raises your blood pressure, increasing strain on your heart and blood vessels.
- **Lipid Imbalances**: High cortisol lowers "good" HDL cholesterol and raises "bad" LDL cholesterol, a dangerous mix for heart health.

3. Muscle Loss and Weakness

Cortisol is catabolic, meaning it breaks down tissues to release energy. Over time, this can lead to muscle loss, leaving you feeling weaker and more fatigued.

- **The Science**: Prolonged cortisol elevation can reduce protein synthesis, the process your body uses to repair and build muscles.
- **Daily Impact**: You might notice reduced stamina, slower recovery after workouts, or even an overall sense of frailty.

4. Weakened Immune System

Cortisol suppresses immune function, making your body less effective at fighting off infections. It's no coincidence that people under chronic stress often find themselves catching colds or battling illnesses more frequently.

- **Autoimmune Risks**: Paradoxically, long-term stress can also overstimulate certain parts of your immune system, increasing the risk of autoimmune diseases.

5. Mental Health Struggles

Your brain isn't immune to cortisol's effects. Chronic elevation is strongly linked to anxiety, depression, and memory problems.

- **Memory and Focus**: High cortisol levels shrink the hippocampus, the part of the brain responsible for learning and memory.

- **Mood Swings**: The constant flood of stress hormones can make you feel irritable, overwhelmed, or even hopeless.

Early Warning Signs of Cortisol Imbalance

Recognizing the early signs of cortisol imbalance can help you take action before the long-term effects set in. These symptoms might seem unrelated at first, but they often point back to elevated cortisol.

Physical Symptoms
- **Persistent Weight Gain**: Especially around your belly, despite maintaining a healthy diet and exercise routine.
- **Fatigue That Won't Quit**: Feeling tired no matter how much sleep you get, or experiencing energy crashes in the afternoon.
- **Digestive Issues**: Bloating, constipation, or diarrhea due to cortisol's impact on gut health.
- **Frequent Illness**: Regularly catching colds, or taking longer than usual to recover.
- **Skin Problems**: Acne, eczema, or slow wound healing caused by immune suppression.

Emotional and Mental Clues
- **Difficulty Concentrating**: Feeling scatterbrained or forgetful.
- **Increased Anxiety**: A constant sense of worry or unease.
- **Mood Swings**: Quick shifts from irritable to sad, or feeling emotionally drained.
- **Sleep Disturbances**: Trouble falling or staying asleep, or waking up feeling unrested.

Behavioral Patterns

- **Cravings for Comfort Foods**: An overwhelming desire for sweets, carbs, or salty snacks.
- **Overworking and Underresting**: Feeling the need to always "be on," even when you're exhausted.

A Real-Life Example: The Impact of Ignoring the Signs

Meet Katherine, a 42-year-old teacher and mother of two. For years, she brushed off her symptoms as "just life." She'd gained 15 pounds despite eating healthy, her sleep was restless, and she found herself snapping at her kids over minor things. After a particularly bad cold that lasted three weeks, Sarah decided to see her doctor.

Blood tests revealed elevated cortisol levels, and further evaluation showed early signs of metabolic syndrome. Sarah's story isn't unique—many people don't realize how much stress has affected their health until it's too late. But with lifestyle changes and a targeted plan (like the one in this book), Sarah was able to reset her cortisol and regain her energy and focus.

How to Test for Cortisol Imbalance

If you suspect cortisol is out of control, consider speaking with a healthcare provider about testing. Here are some common methods:

1. **Saliva Tests**: These measure cortisol levels at different times of the day to see if your natural rhythm is disrupted.
2. **Blood Tests**: Often done in the morning when cortisol is naturally highest.
3. **Urine Tests**: Provide a 24-hour snapshot of cortisol levels.

Understanding your levels can help tailor your approach to managing stress and restoring balance.

Your Body's Cry for Balance

High cortisol doesn't happen overnight, and neither do its effects. But the beauty of the human body is its ability to heal and adapt. Recognizing the cost of imbalance—and the signs that something's off—is the first step to reclaiming your health.

In the next chapter, we'll dive into the foods and nutrients that naturally support cortisol balance, showing you how small changes to your diet can have a big impact. Remember, this journey isn't about perfection—it's about progress. With the right tools and knowledge, you can reset your cortisol levels and feel like yourself again.

Part 2: Foods That Heal – Eating Your Way to Hormonal Harmony

CHAPTER 4
THE ANTI-CORTISOL PANTRY

Your pantry isn't just a collection of ingredients; it's your first line of defense against the stress hormone cortisol. The foods you eat play a massive role in either fueling or calming the stress response. By stocking up on cortisol-balancing staples and avoiding triggers, you can create meals that support your body's hormonal rhythm and help you feel more balanced and energized. Let's dive into the must-haves and the must-avoids to transform your kitchen into a sanctuary for your health.

The Top 10 Cortisol-Balancing Foods

1. **Sweet Potatoes**
   Sweet potatoes are rich in complex carbohydrates, which help stabilize blood sugar levels. Balanced blood sugar means your body is less likely to overproduce cortisol in response to dips and spikes.

2. **Avocados**
   Packed with healthy monounsaturated fats, avocados are fantastic for supporting brain health and reducing inflammation, both of which are key to keeping cortisol in check.

3. **Salmon**
   Rich in omega-3 fatty acids, salmon has anti-inflammatory properties that counteract the damaging effects of chronic stress. Omega-3s also help regulate mood by interacting with cortisol and serotonin pathways.

4. **Leafy Greens**
   Spinach, kale, and Swiss chard are loaded with magnesium, a mineral

known for its ability to relax muscles and calm the nervous system. Magnesium deficiency is closely linked to elevated cortisol levels.

5. **Blueberries**
These tiny powerhouses are rich in antioxidants, which help neutralize oxidative stress caused by high cortisol. They're also a natural source of vitamin C, another stress-busting nutrient.

6. **Eggs**
Eggs are a fantastic source of high-quality protein, which supports hormone production and helps stabilize energy levels throughout the day.

7. **Pumpkin Seeds**
These seeds are an excellent snack option for keeping cortisol levels steady. They're high in magnesium, zinc, and tryptophan, which collectively support relaxation and reduce stress.

8. **Greek Yogurt**
Packed with probiotics, Greek yogurt promotes gut health—a crucial factor in managing stress and cortisol. An imbalanced gut can send stress signals to the brain, perpetuating high cortisol.

9. **Chamomile Tea**
This calming tea has been shown to reduce stress and promote better sleep. A warm cup in the evening can help reset your cortisol curve, which should naturally taper off at night.

10. **Dark Chocolate (70% or Higher)**
Dark chocolate in moderation can reduce cortisol levels by triggering the release of endorphins and providing antioxidants. Just be mindful of portion sizes and avoid added sugars.

Building Your Anti-Cortisol Pantry

To start your journey, you need the right tools—and by tools, we mean the essentials that should fill your shelves. Here's what to stock up on and why each ingredient deserves a spot in your pantry.

Pantry Staples

- **Whole Grains**: Oats, quinoa, and brown rice are great sources of complex carbs that stabilize energy levels and support a calm cortisol curve.
- **Nuts and Seeds**: Almonds, walnuts, chia seeds, and flaxseeds are nutrient-dense options loaded with healthy fats and magnesium.
- **Herbs and Spices**: Turmeric, cinnamon, and ginger have anti-inflammatory and cortisol-lowering properties.
- **Legumes**: Lentils, chickpeas, and black beans provide plant-based protein and fiber to support gut health and energy stability.
- **Olive Oil**: A heart-healthy fat, olive oil is an anti-inflammatory staple for cooking or drizzling over salads.
- **Fermented Foods**: Sauerkraut, kimchi, and miso promote a healthy gut microbiome, indirectly aiding cortisol regulation.
- **Coconut Milk**: A versatile ingredient for creamy soups and smoothies that also contains healthy fats to stabilize hormones.
- **Green Tea**: Rich in L-theanine, a compound that promotes relaxation and reduces stress.

Fresh Essentials

- **Seasonal Fruits**: Apples, oranges, and bananas for natural sweetness and antioxidants.
- **Veggies**: Broccoli, carrots, and bell peppers for their high vitamin C content.
- **Lean Proteins**: Chicken, turkey, and tofu to support muscle maintenance and steady energy levels.

Foods to Avoid

Just as important as what you include is what you leave out. Some foods can act as stress triggers, increasing cortisol production and making it harder for your body to reset.

1. **Refined Sugars**
   High-sugar foods like candies, pastries, and sweetened drinks cause blood sugar spikes, which lead to a reactive rise in cortisol.

2. **Processed Foods**
   Chips, frozen dinners, and other ultra-processed items often contain unhealthy fats and high levels of sodium, which can exacerbate stress on the body.

3. **Caffeine**
   While coffee has its perks, overconsumption can spike cortisol, especially if you're already stressed. Try limiting intake to one cup a day or swapping it for green tea.

4. **Alcohol**
   While it might feel like a stress reliever, alcohol disrupts sleep and interferes with your body's ability to regulate cortisol.

5. **Artificial Sweeteners**
   These can trick your body into releasing stress hormones while providing zero nutritional value.

6. **Fried Foods**
   These are high in trans fats, which promote inflammation and disrupt hormonal balance.

Making It Actionable

A pantry transformation doesn't have to happen overnight. Start small by swapping out one or two stress-triggering ingredients for cortisol-friendly alternatives. Here are some easy swaps:

Instead Of...	Try This...
Sugary Breakfast Cereals	Oatmeal with fresh berries
White Bread	Sprouted grain bread
Potato Chips	Air-popped popcorn with olive oil
Soda	Sparkling water with a splash of citrus
Coffee	Matcha or herbal tea

A Sample Shopping List

To help you get started, here's a basic shopping list to fill your pantry and fridge with cortisol-friendly options:

Fruits and Vegetables
- Blueberries, oranges, and bananas
- Spinach, broccoli, and bell peppers

Proteins and Dairy
- Eggs, chicken, and salmon
- Greek yogurt and unsweetened almond milk

Pantry Essentials
- Brown rice, oats, and quinoa
- Olive oil, coconut milk, and raw nuts

Extras
- Dark chocolate (70% or higher)
- Chamomile and green teas

Bringing It All Together

Your pantry is the foundation for your cortisol detox journey. By stocking up on nutrient-dense, stress-reducing foods and cutting out the culprits that elevate cortisol, you're giving your body the tools it needs to thrive.

Remember, the key is balance—not perfection. Even small changes to your diet can make a big difference in how you feel. As you start incorporating these foods into your daily meals, you'll likely notice improved energy, mood, and focus.

In the next chapter, we'll explore how to turn these ingredients into delicious, stress-busting recipes that fit seamlessly into your lifestyle.

CHAPTER 5

RECIPES FOR RELAXATION

Quick and easy meal ideas tailored to balance blood sugar and lower inflammation.

When life gets hectic, the meals you eat should provide more than just fuel—they should help calm your body and mind. This chapter is all about quick, easy recipes that support cortisol balance, reduce inflammation, and keep your blood sugar steady. These dishes are not only nourishing but also packed with sensory appeal: warm, soothing, aromatic, and bursting with flavor. Let's dive into breakfasts, snacks, and drinks designed to comfort your body and keep stress at bay.

Breakfast: Start Your Day Calm and Balanced

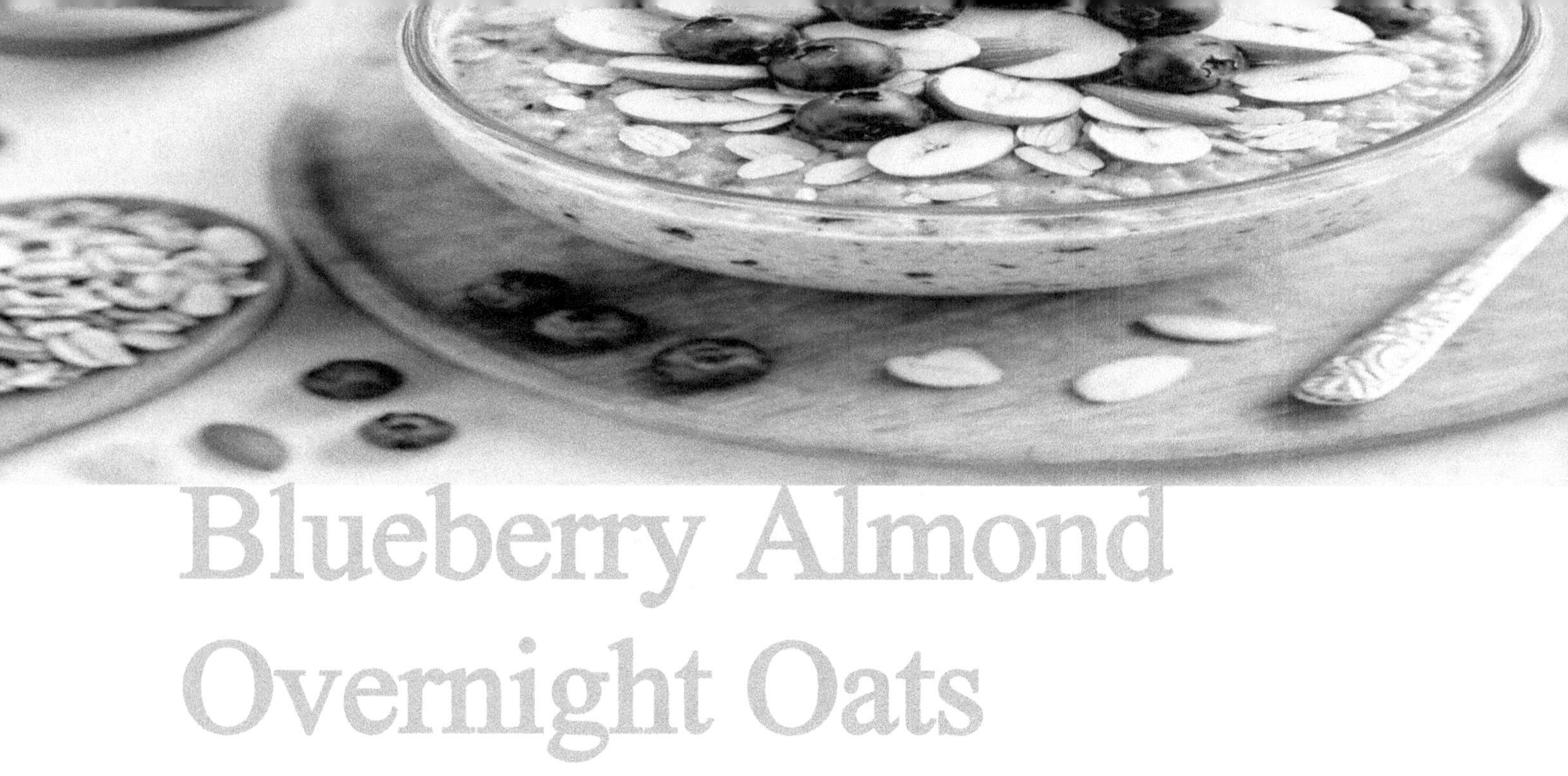

Blueberry Almond Overnight Oats

INGREDIENTS:

- ½ cup rolled oats
- 1 tablespoon chia seeds
- ¾ cup unsweetened almond milk
- ½ cup fresh blueberries
- 1 tablespoon almond butter
- 1 teaspoon honey

INSTRUCTIONS:

- Combine oats, chia seeds, and almond milk in a jar or bowl. Stir well.
- Top with blueberries, almond butter, and honey. Cover and refrigerate overnight.
- Enjoy chilled or warmed slightly in the morning.

Prep Time: 5 minutes
Cook Time: 0 minutes

Nutritional Info: 240 calories, 7g protein, 10g fat, 30g carbs

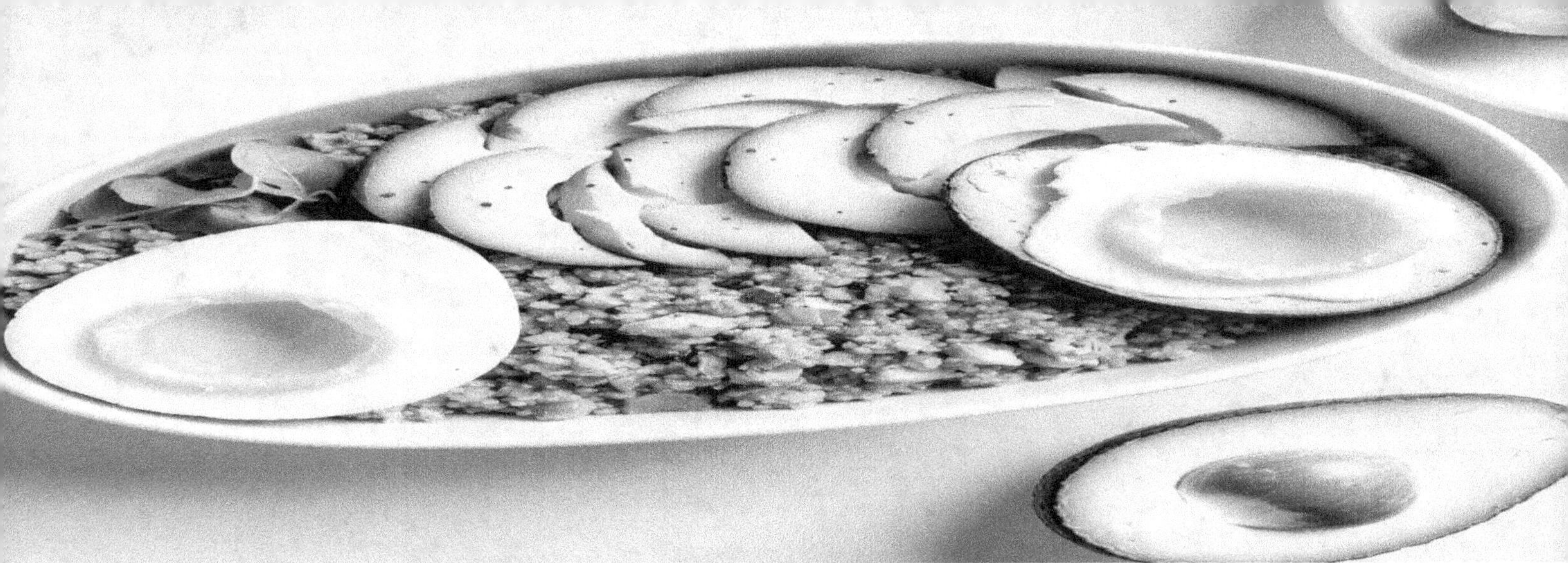

Avocado and Egg Breakfast Bowl

INGREDIENTS:

- 1 ripe avocado
- 2 boiled eggs
- ½ cup cooked quinoa
- 1 teaspoon olive oil
- Salt and pepper to taste

INSTRUCTIONS:

- Slice the avocado and eggs.
- Arrange avocado, eggs, and quinoa in a bowl. Drizzle with olive oil.
- Sprinkle with salt and pepper. Serve immediately.

Prep Time: 10 minutes
Cook Time: 10 minutes
Nutritional Info: 290 calories, 13g protein, 18g fat, 20g carbs

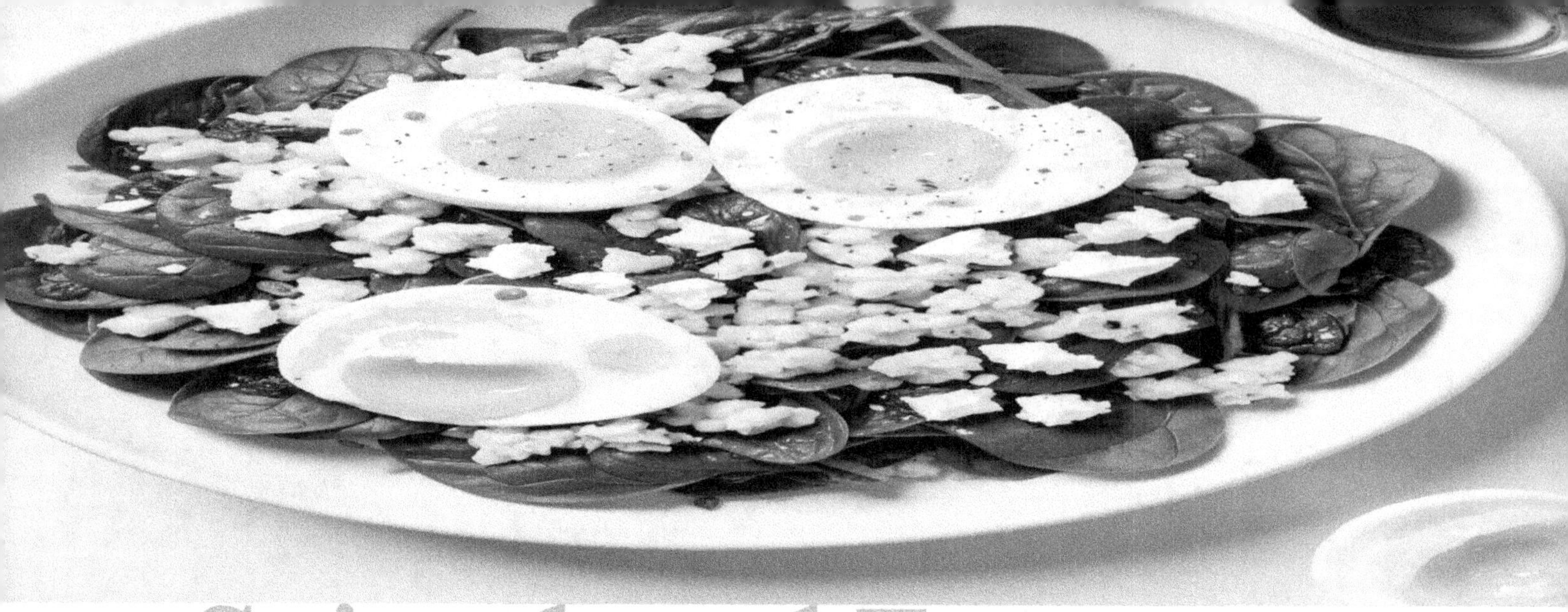

Spinach and Feta Scramble

INGREDIENTS:

- 2 large eggs
- ½ cup fresh spinach
- 2 tablespoons crumbled feta cheese
- 1 teaspoon olive oil
- Salt and pepper to taste

INSTRUCTIONS:

- Heat olive oil in a skillet over medium heat.
- Add spinach and cook until wilted.
- Whisk eggs, pour into the skillet, and scramble until cooked through.
- Top with feta cheese and season with salt and pepper.

Prep Time: 5 minutes
Cook Time: 5 minutes

Nutritional Info: 190 calories, 13g protein, 14g fat, 3g carbs

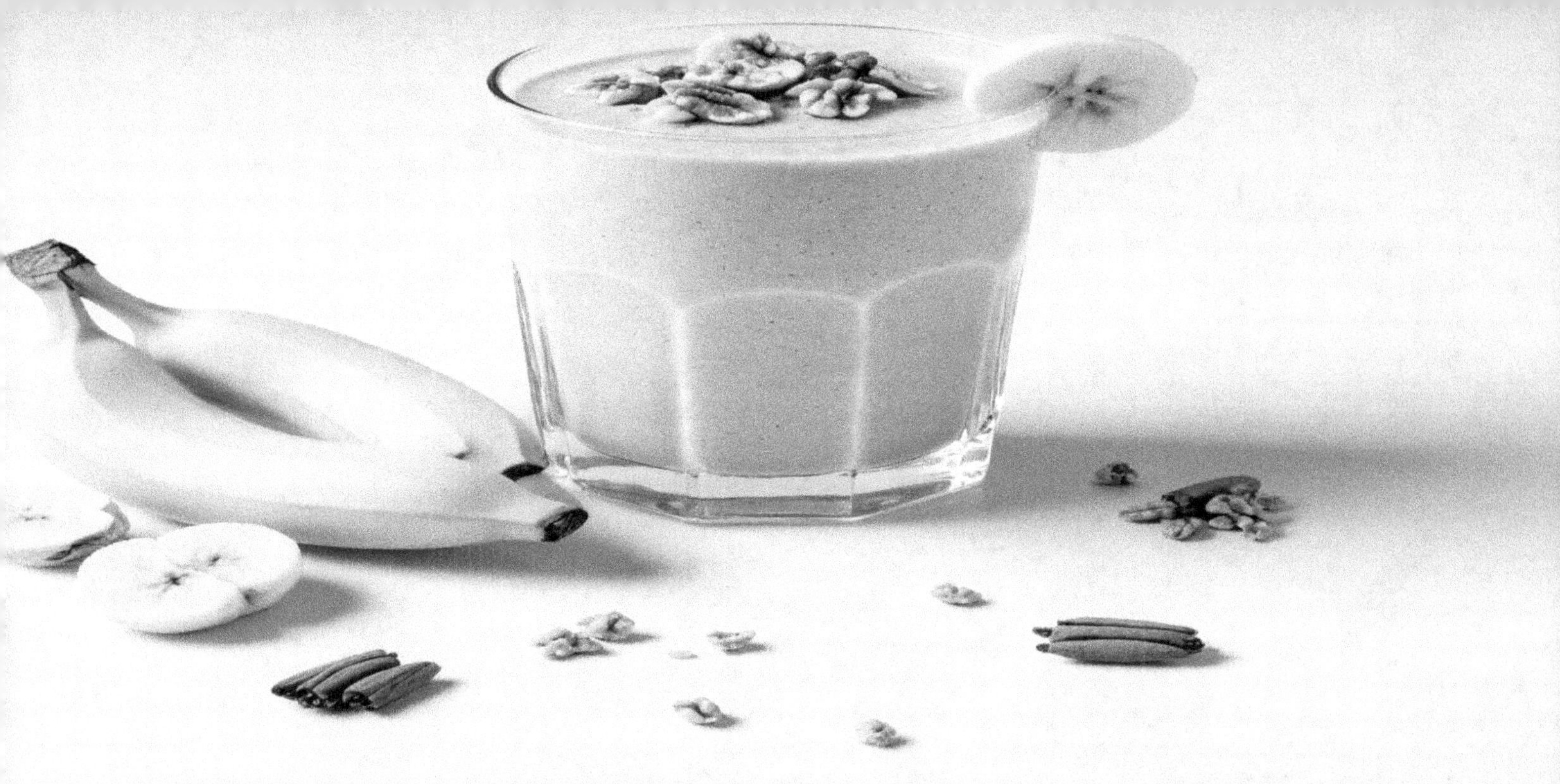

Banana Walnut Smoothie

INGREDIENTS:
- 1 ripe banana
- 1 tablespoon walnuts
- 1 cup unsweetened oat milk
- 1 teaspoon cinnamon

INSTRUCTIONS:
- Blend all ingredients until smooth.
- Pour into a glass and enjoy immediately.

Prep Time: 5 minutes
Cook Time: 0 minutes
Nutritional Info: 210 calories, 4g protein, 8g fat, 34g carbs

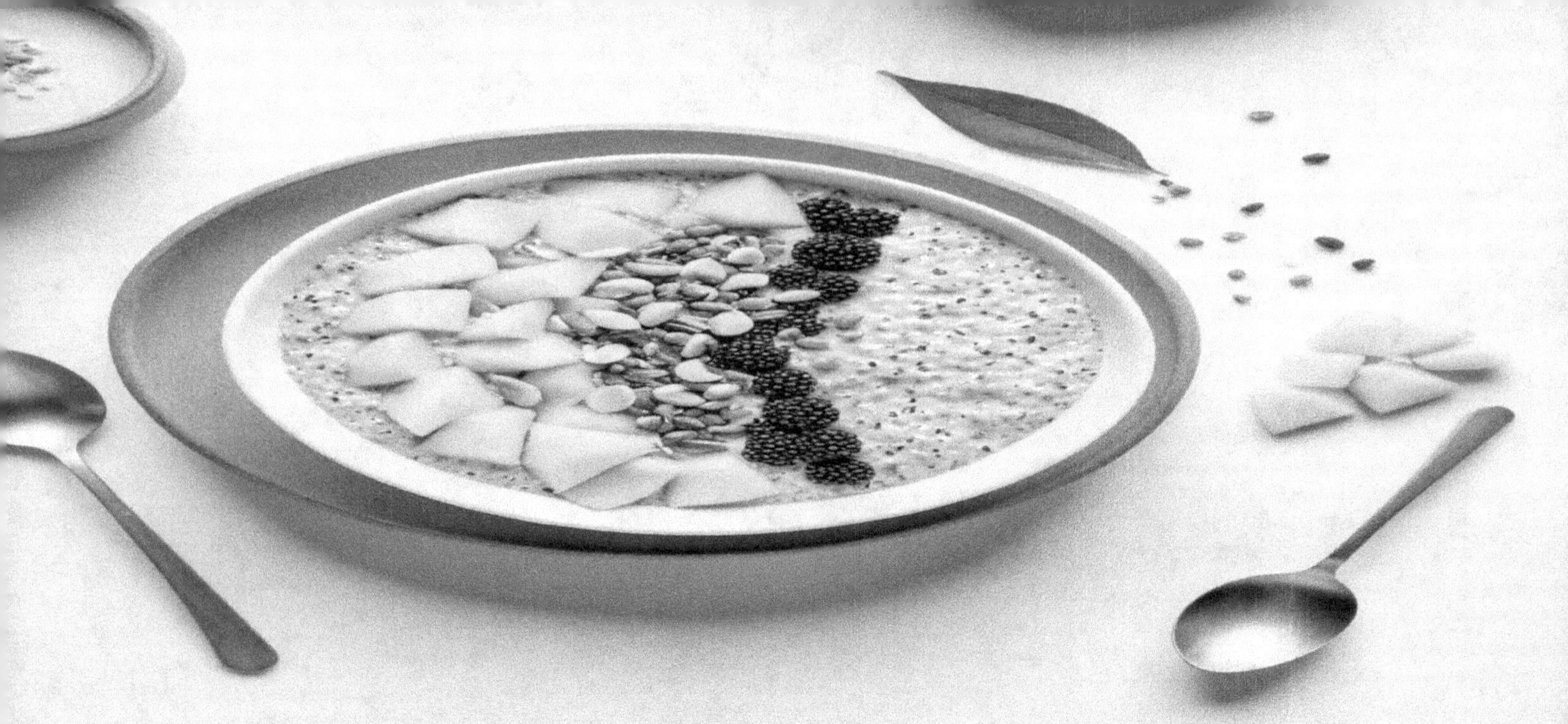

Chia Pudding with Mango

INGREDIENTS:

- 3 tablespoons chia seeds
- 1 cup unsweetened coconut milk
- ½ cup diced fresh mango

INSTRUCTIONS:

- Mix chia seeds and coconut milk in a jar. Stir well.
- Let it sit for at least 4 hours or overnight in the fridge.
- Top with diced mango before serving.

Prep Time: 5 minutes
Cook Time: 0 minutes (4 hours chilling time)

Nutritional Info: 180 calories, 5g protein, 9g fat, 20g carbs

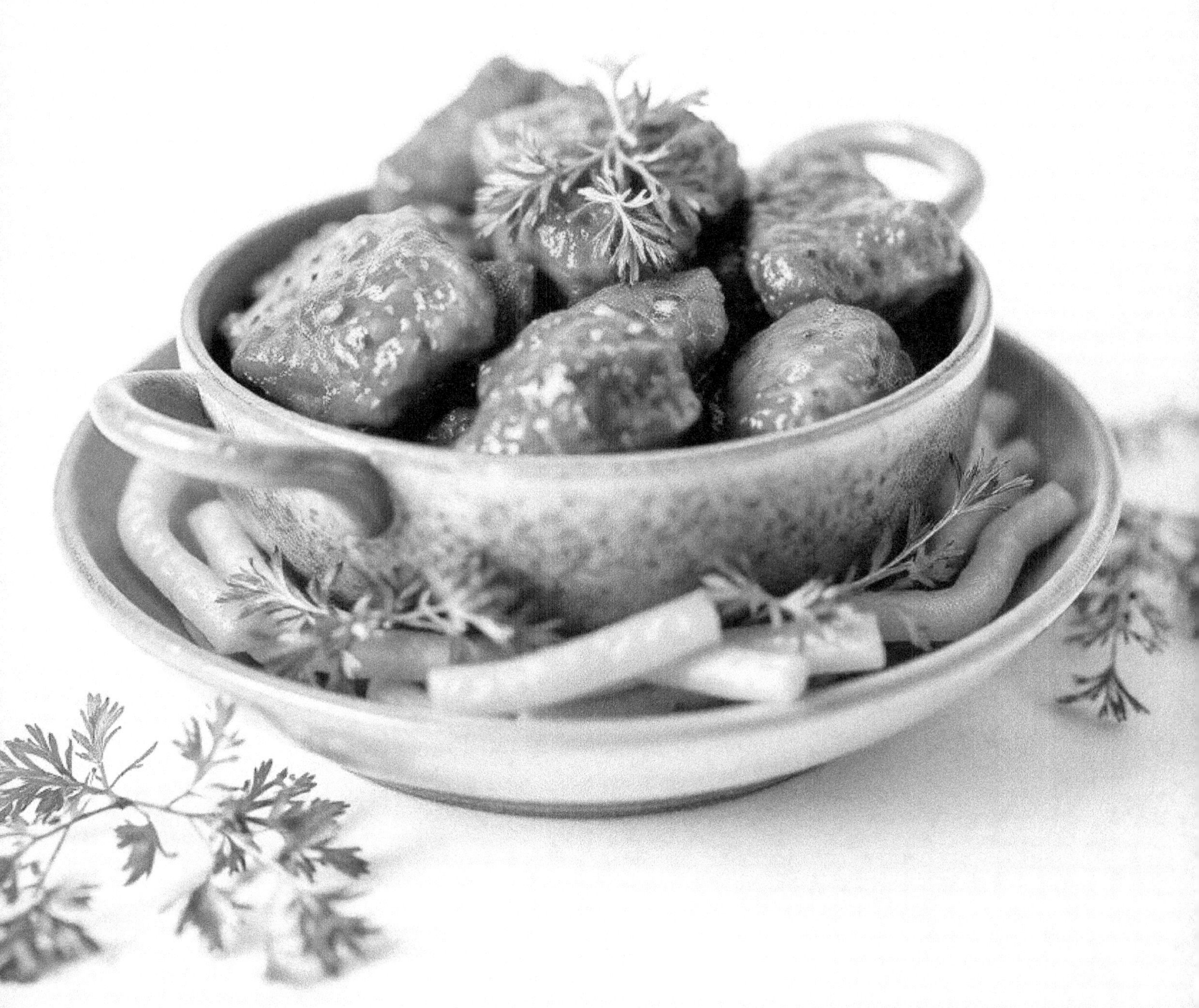

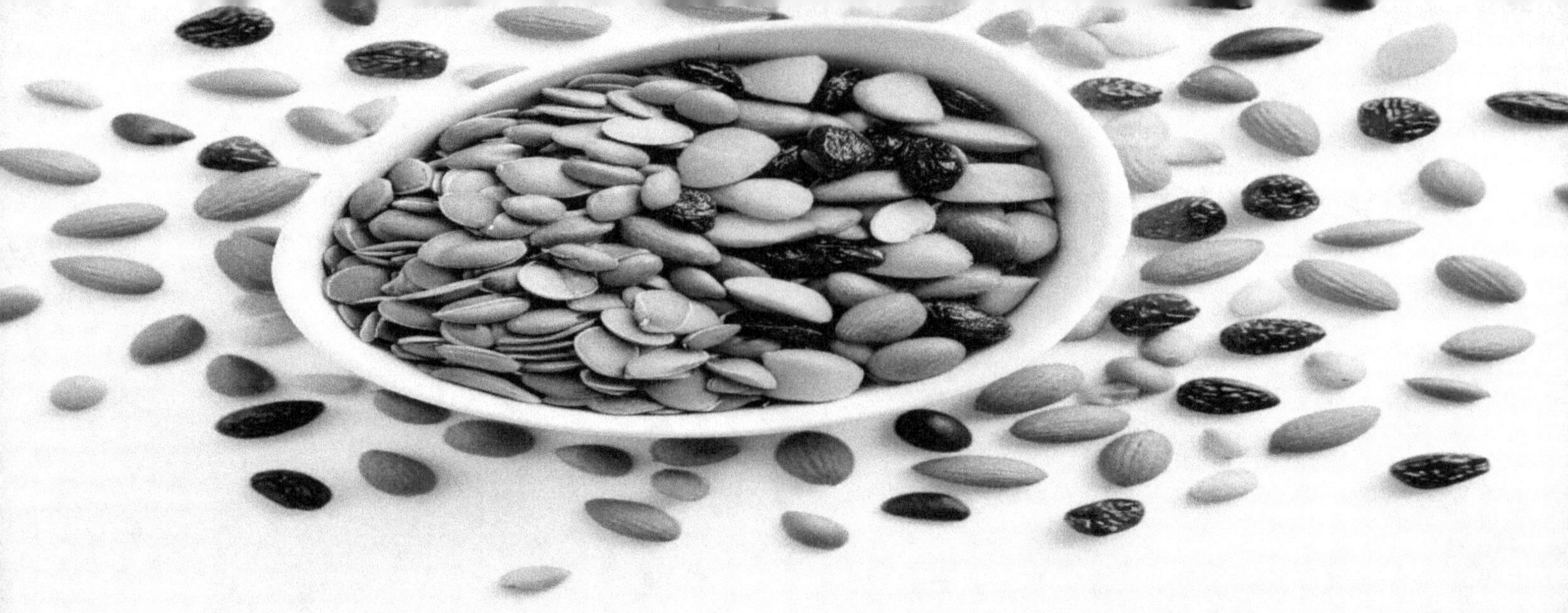

Pumpkin Seed Trail Mix

INGREDIENTS:

- ½ cup pumpkin seeds
- ¼ cup dried cranberries
- ¼ cup dark chocolate chips (70% or higher)
- ¼ cup almonds

INSTRUCTIONS:

- Mix all ingredients in a bowl. Store in an airtight container.

Prep Time: 5 minutes
Cook Time: 0 minutes

Nutritional Info: 200 calories, 6g protein, 12g fat, 18g carbs

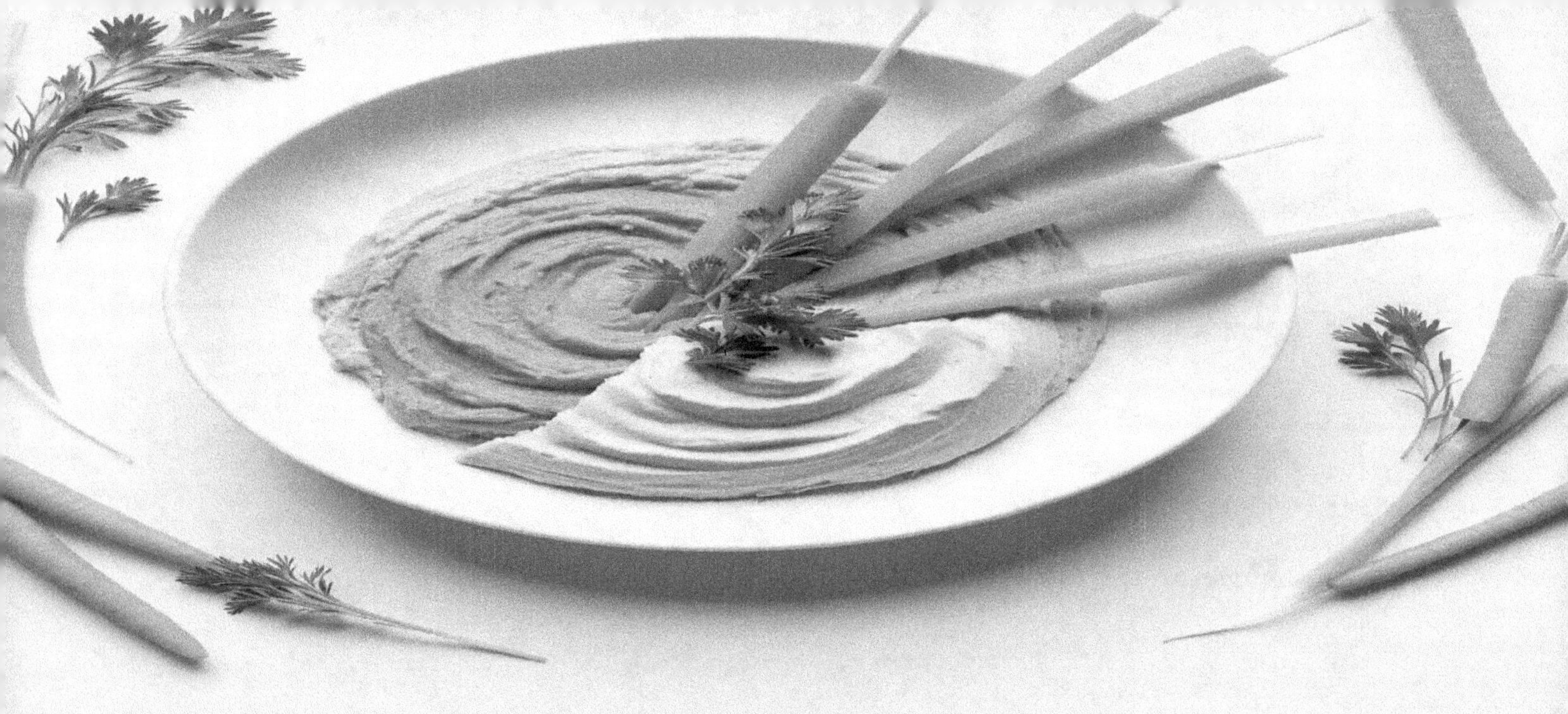

Carrot Sticks with Hummus

INGREDIENTS:

- 1 cup carrot sticks
- 2 tablespoons hummus

INSTRUCTIONS:

- Serve carrot sticks with hummus on the side for dipping.

Prep Time: 5 minutes
Cook Time: 0 minutes

Nutritional Info: 120 calories, 3g protein, 7g fat, 10g carbs

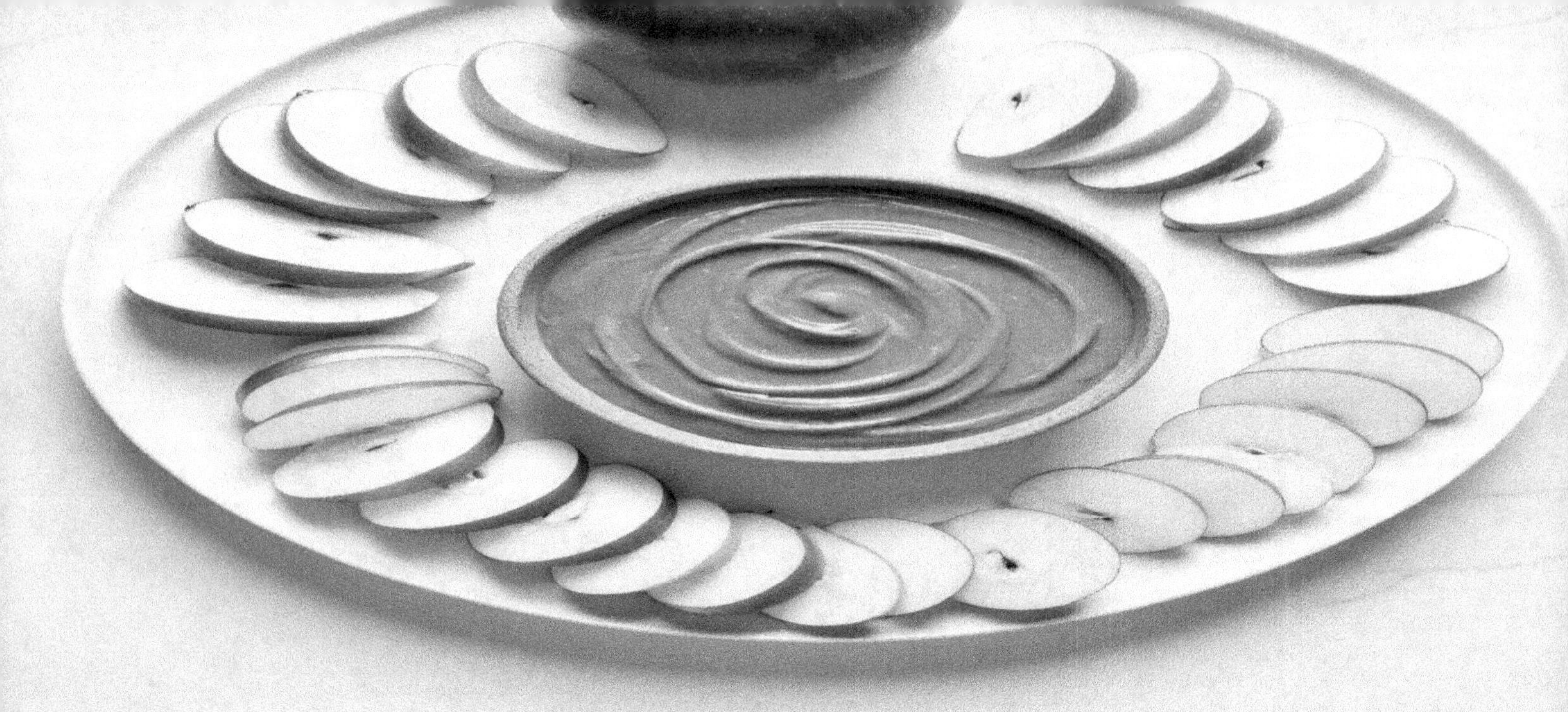

Apple Slices with Almond Butter

INGREDIENTS:

- 1 medium apple, sliced
- 1 tablespoon almond butter

INSTRUCTIONS:

- Spread almond butter on apple slices and enjoy.

Prep Time: 5 minutes
Cook Time: 0 minutes

Nutritional Info: 150 calories, 2g protein, 6g fat, 20g carbs

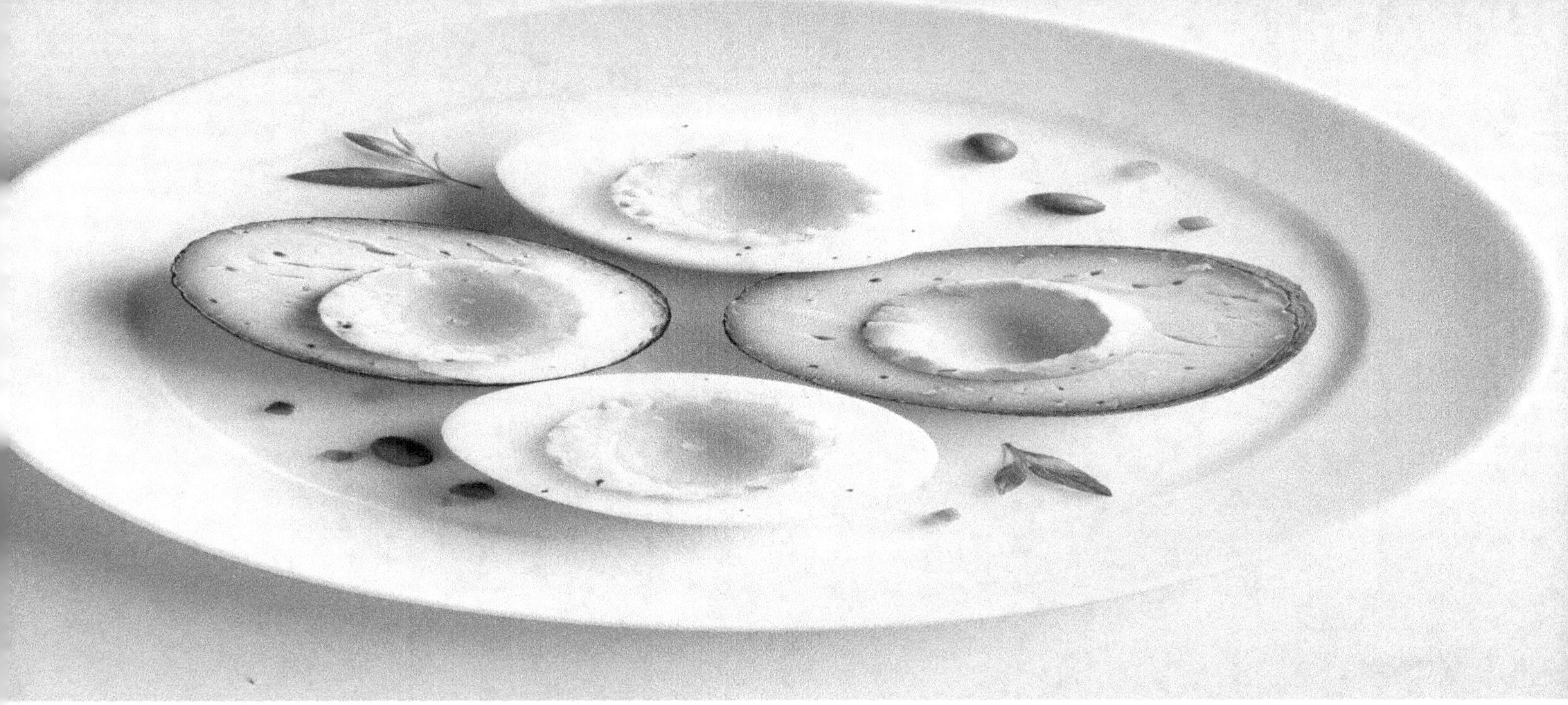

Hard-Boiled Eggs with Avocado

INGREDIENTS:

- 2 hard-boiled eggs
- ½ avocado
- Salt and pepper to taste

INSTRUCTIONS:

- Slice the eggs and avocado.
- Sprinkle with salt and pepper. Serve together.

Prep Time: 5 minutes
Cook Time: 10 minutes

Nutritional Info: 250 calories, 12g protein, 20g fat, 6g carbs

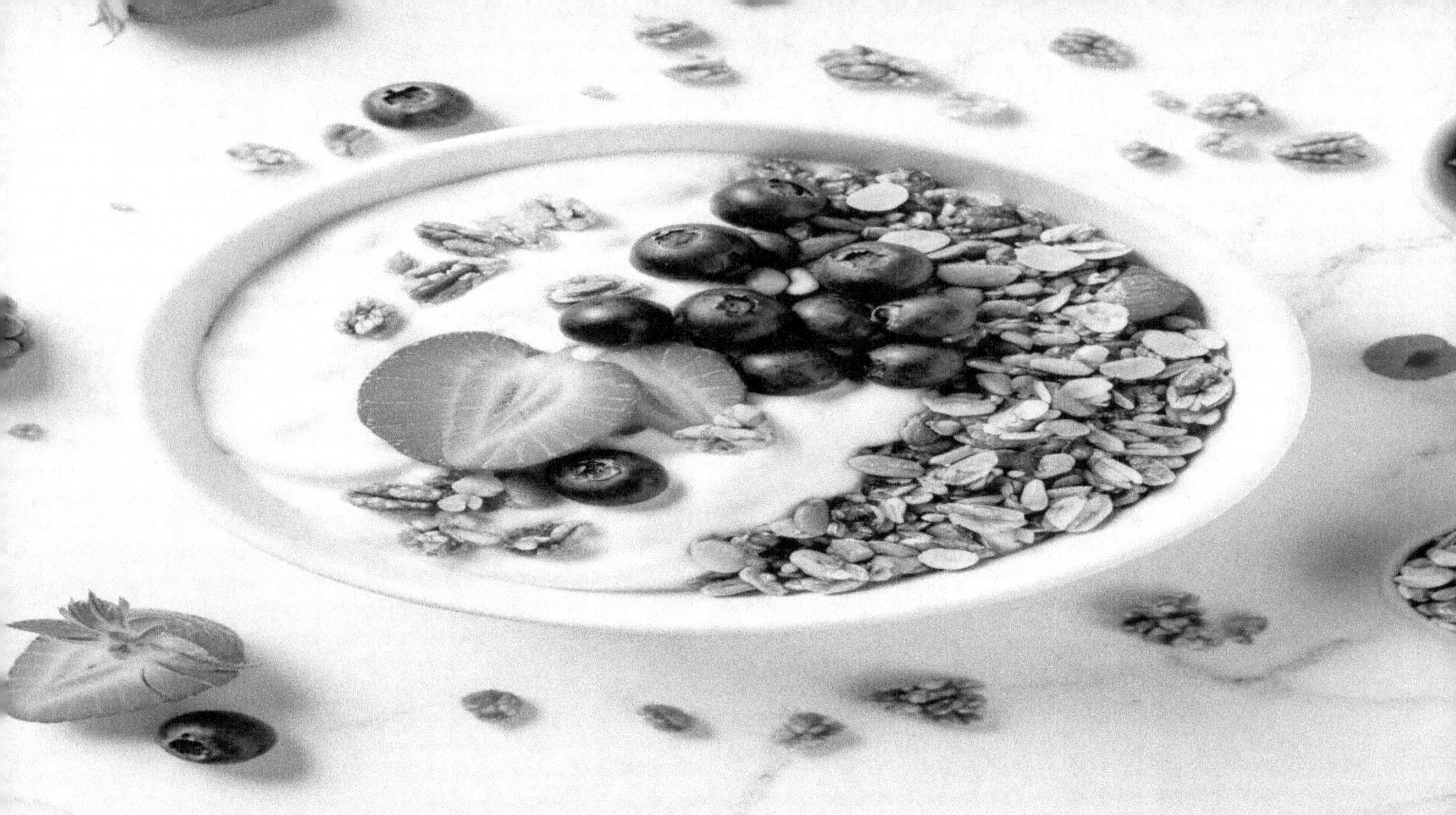

Greek Yogurt Parfait

INGREDIENTS:

- ½ cup Greek yogurt
- ¼ cup granola
- ¼ cup fresh berries

INSTRUCTIONS:

- Layer Greek yogurt, granola, and berries in a bowl or glass.

Prep Time: 5 minutes
Cook Time: 0 minutes

Nutritional Info: 180 calories, 10g protein, 4g fat, 25g carbs

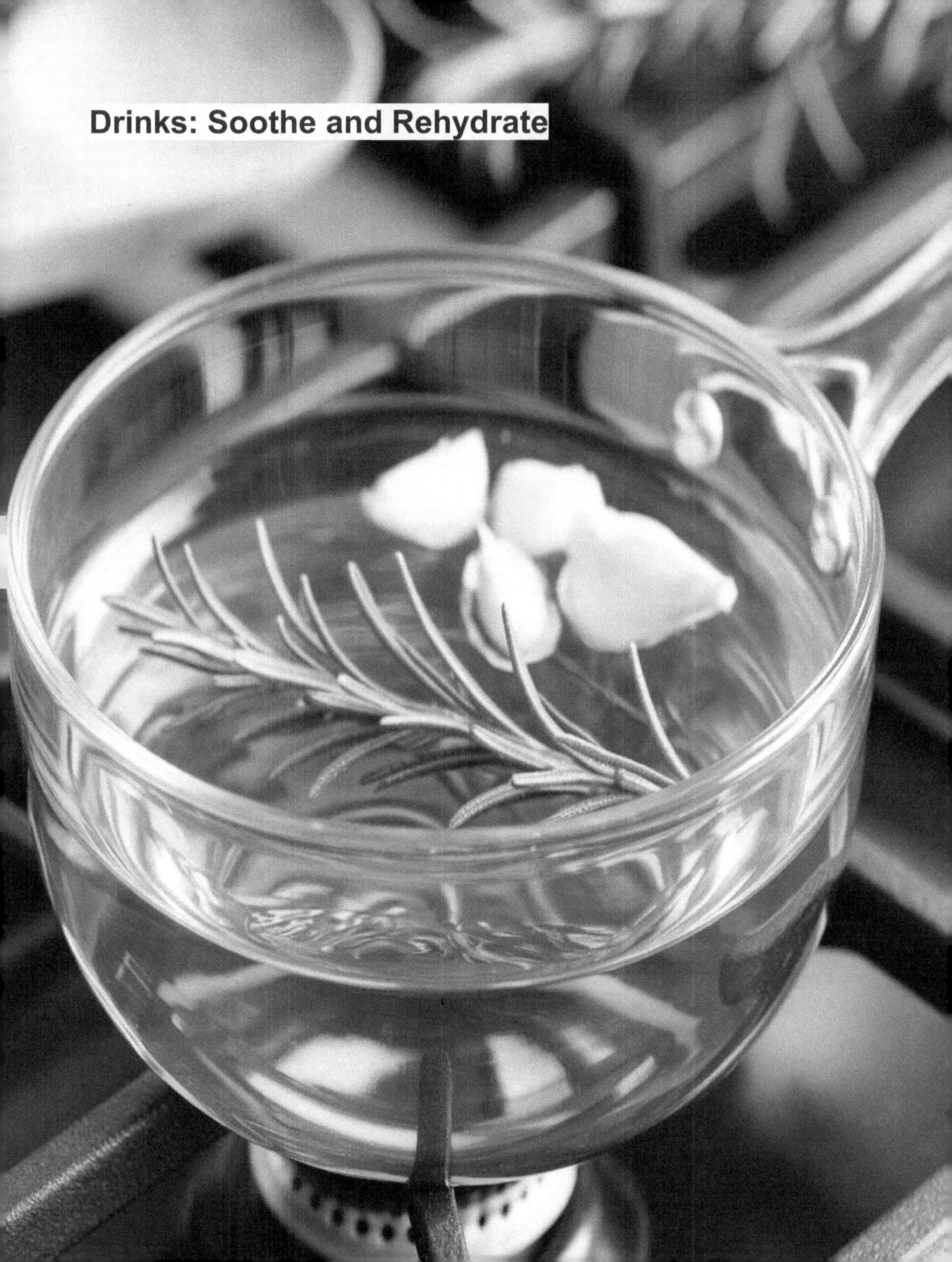
Drinks: Soothe and Rehydrate

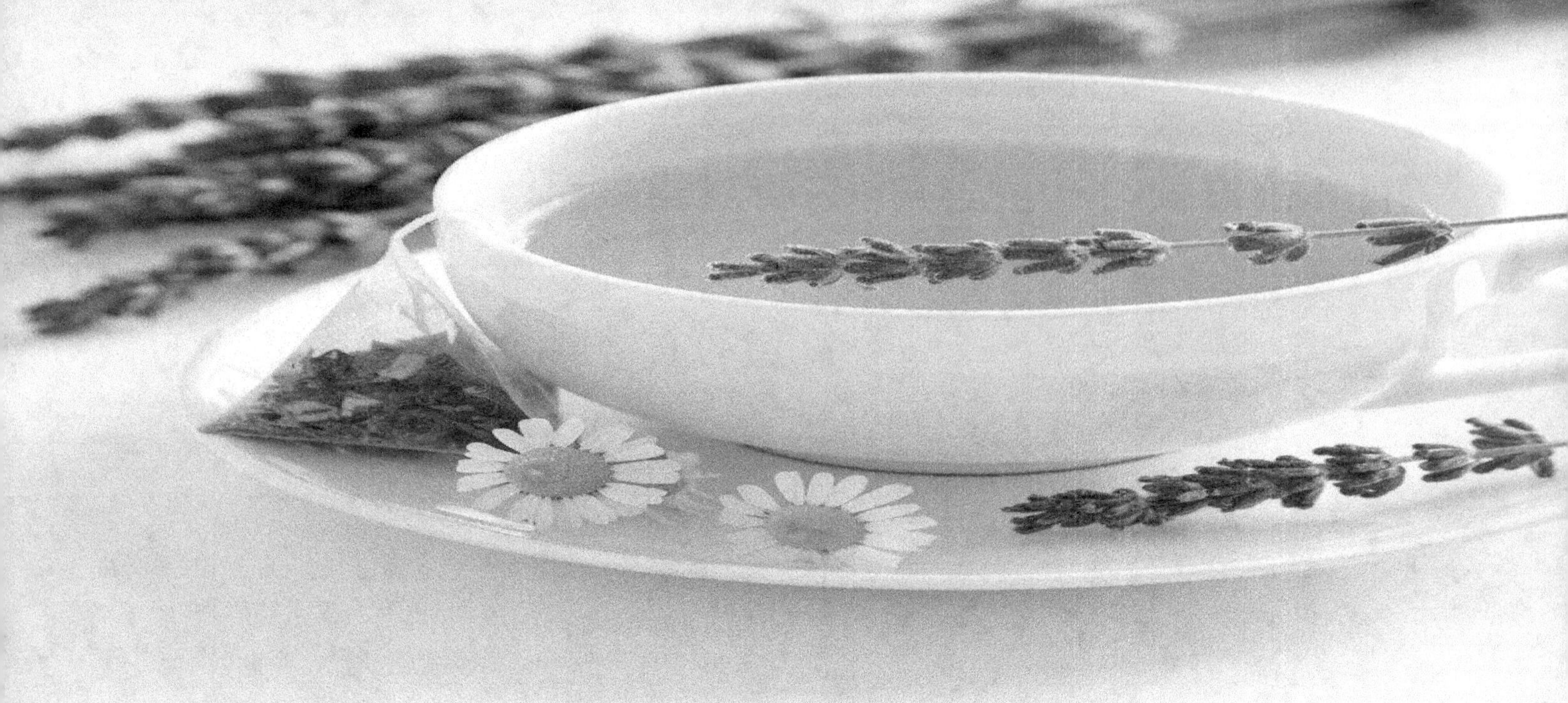

Chamomile Lavender Tea

INGREDIENTS:

- 1 chamomile tea bag
- 1 teaspoon dried lavender
- 1 cup boiling water

INSTRUCTIONS:

- Steep chamomile tea and lavender in boiling water for 5 minutes. Strain and enjoy warm.

Prep Time: 2 minutes
Cook Time: 5 minutes

Nutritional Info: 0 calories, 0g protein, 0g fat, 0g carbs

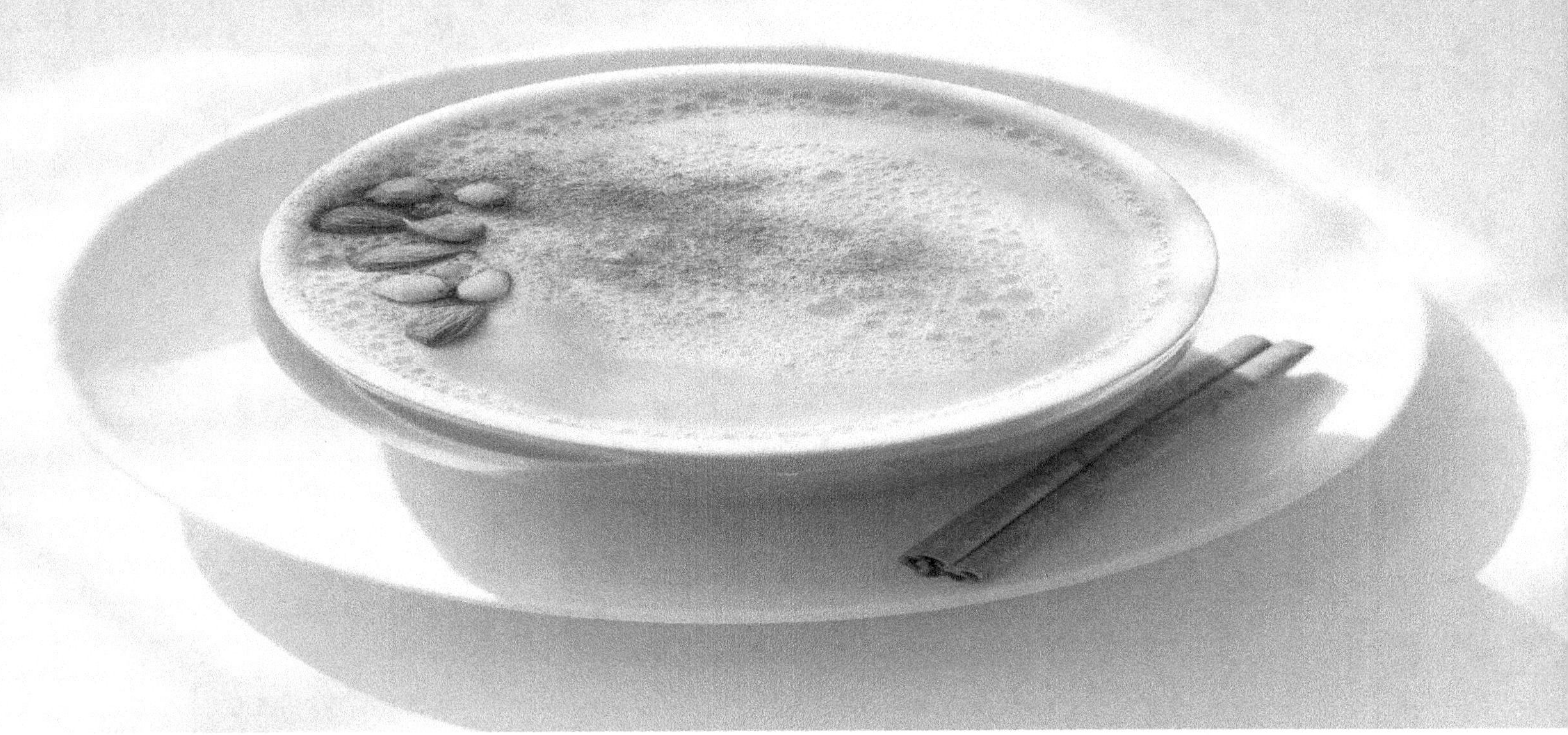

Golden Milk

INGREDIENTS:

- 1 cup unsweetened almond milk
- ½ teaspoon turmeric
- ¼ teaspoon cinnamon
- 1 teaspoon honey

INSTRUCTIONS:

- Heat almond milk in a saucepan. Stir in turmeric, cinnamon, and honey.
- Pour into a mug and enjoy warm.

Prep Time: 2 minutes
Cook Time: 5 minutes

Nutritional Info: 50 calories, 1g protein, 2g fat, 8g carbs

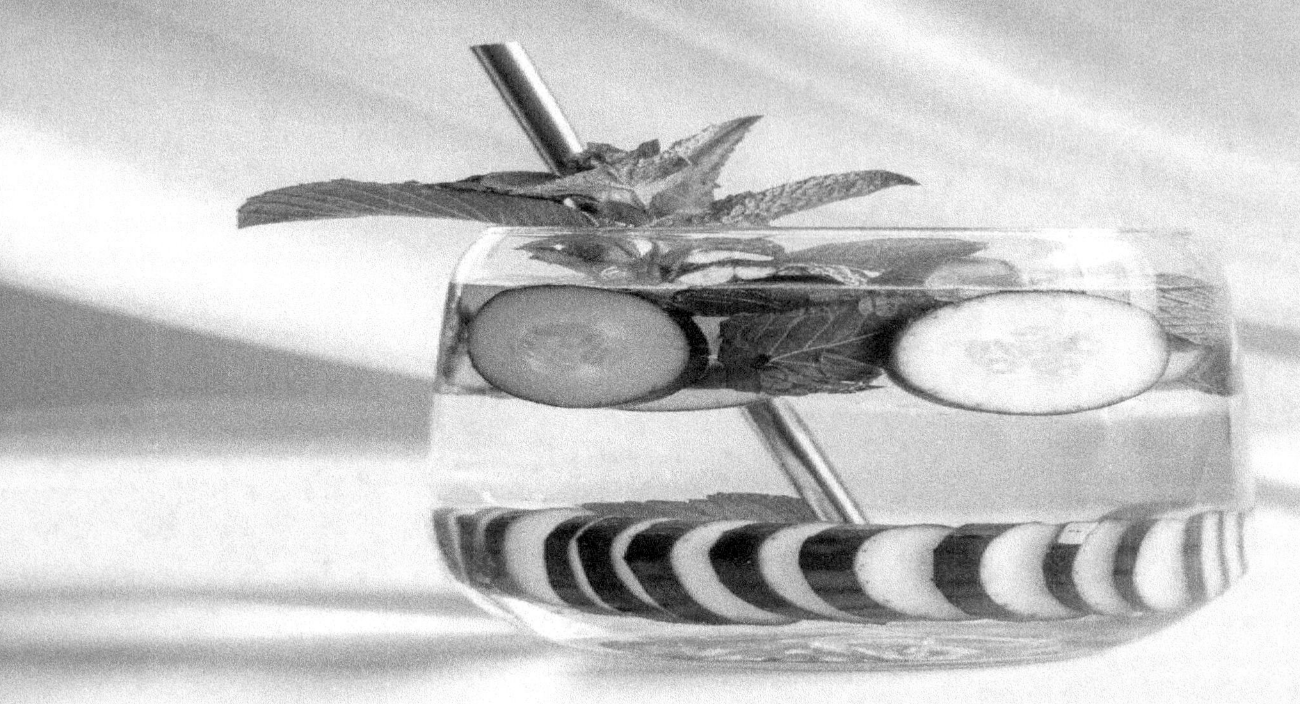

Mint Cucumber Water

INGREDIENTS:

- 1 liter water
- ½ cucumber, sliced
- 10 fresh mint leaves

INSTRUCTIONS:

- Combine all ingredients in a pitcher. Let infuse for 1 hour in the fridge.

Prep Time: 5 minutes
Cook Time: 0 minutes

Nutritional Info: 0 calories, 0g protein, 0g fat, 0g carbs

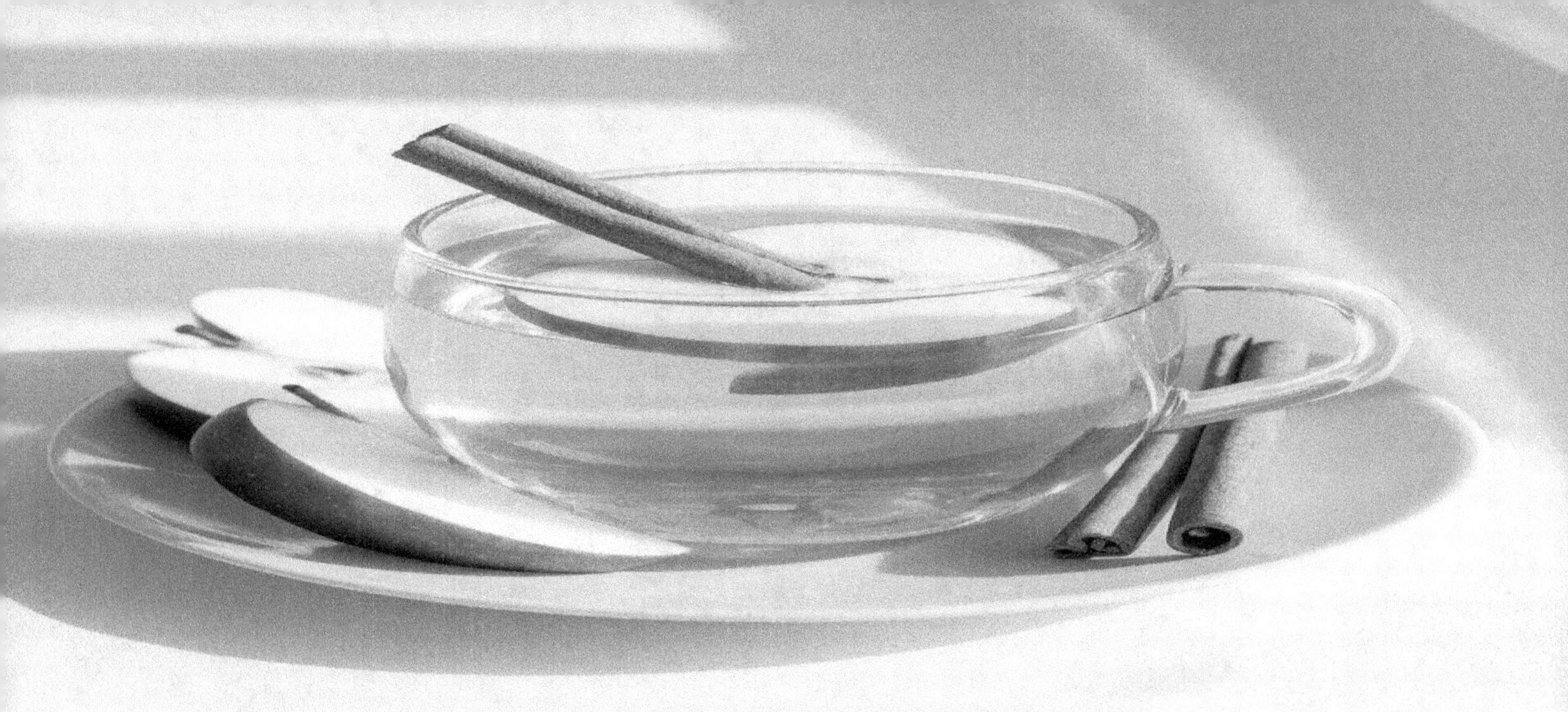

Cinnamon Apple Infusion

INGREDIENTS:
- 1 cup boiling water
- 1 apple slice
- 1 cinnamon stick

INSTRUCTIONS:
- Steep apple slice and cinnamon stick in boiling water for 10 minutes.

Prep Time: 2 minutes
Cook Time: 10 minutes

Nutritional Info: 0 calories, 0g protein, 0g fat, 0g carbs

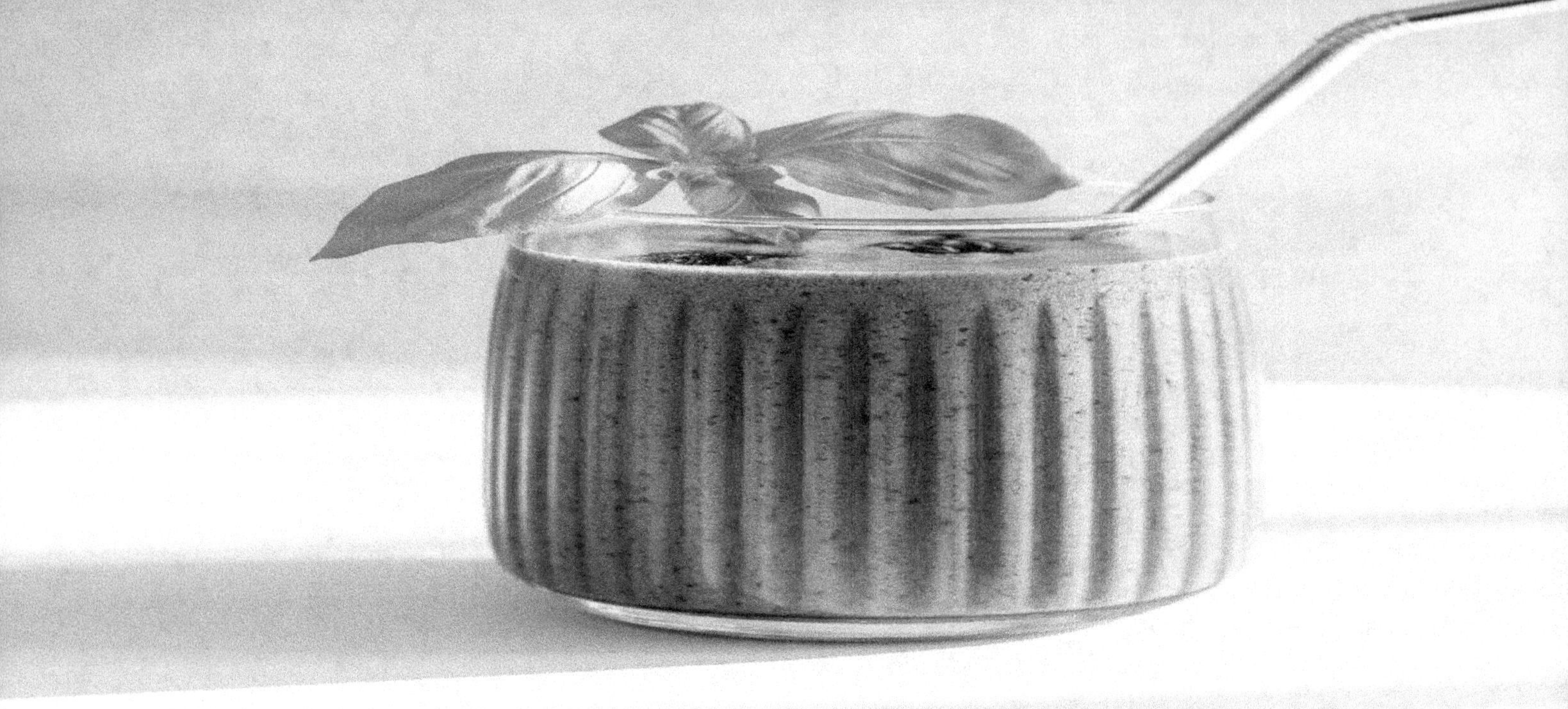

Berry Basil Smoothie

INGREDIENTS:

- 1 cup frozen mixed berries
- 5 fresh basil leaves
- 1 cup unsweetened coconut water

INSTRUCTIONS:

- Blend all ingredients until smooth. Serve chilled.

Prep Time: 5 minutes
Cook Time: 0 minutes

Nutritional Info: 70 calories, 1g protein, 0g fat, 18g carbs

CHAPTER 6

NUTRITIONAL HACKS FOR STRESS RELIEF

Stress can sneak into our lives in subtle ways, but the good news is that the right foods, supplements, and hydration strategies can make a huge difference in how our bodies handle it. This chapter is all about practical nutritional tools—adaptogens, superfoods, supplements, and hydration tips—that can help keep cortisol levels in check. Let's break it down in a way that feels easy to implement, even on your busiest days.

Adaptogens: Nature's Stress Fighters

Adaptogens are natural substances that help your body adapt to stress. They work by supporting your adrenal glands, which produce cortisol, to maintain balance during times of physical or mental strain. Here are a few adaptogens worth exploring:

1. Ashwagandha

- **Why It Works**: Ashwagandha has been shown to lower cortisol levels and improve overall resilience to stress. It's particularly helpful for people dealing with chronic stress or sleep disturbances.
- **How to Use It**: Add ashwagandha powder to smoothies, teas, or golden milk. Capsules are another convenient option.
- **Tip**: Pair it with warm drinks for a soothing evening ritual.

2. Rhodiola Rosea

- **Why It Works**: Rhodiola helps reduce mental fatigue and boosts energy levels, making it a great choice for those feeling drained by stress.
- **How to Use It**: Mix rhodiola extract into herbal teas or sprinkle it into morning oatmeal. Capsules are available for a more concentrated dose.

3. Holy Basil (Tulsi)
- **Why It Works**: Holy basil is known for its calming properties and ability to lower cortisol. It also supports immunity, which can weaken under stress.
- **How to Use It**: Brew it as tea or incorporate fresh tulsi leaves into soups and salads.

4. Maca Root
- **Why It Works**: Maca root balances hormones and boosts energy without spiking cortisol. It's also rich in nutrients like vitamin C and iron.
- **How to Use It**: Blend maca powder into coffee, smoothies, or baked goods for a nutty, earthy flavor.

Supplements for Stress Relief

While food is the foundation, certain supplements can provide targeted support for cortisol management:

1. Magnesium
- **Why It Works**: Magnesium plays a key role in regulating the nervous system and can help reduce cortisol spikes caused by stress.
- **Sources**: Look for magnesium glycinate or citrate supplements. Natural sources include spinach, almonds, and dark chocolate.

2. Omega-3 Fatty Acids
- **Why It Works**: Omega-3s combat inflammation and support brain health, both of which can suffer under prolonged stress.
- **Sources**: Fish oil supplements are an excellent source, but you can also get omega-3s from fatty fish like salmon and plant-based options like chia seeds.

3. B Vitamins
- **Why They Work**: B vitamins, especially B6 and B12, support adrenal function and energy production. Stress can deplete these vitamins, so replenishing them is crucial.
- **Sources**: Look for B-complex supplements or eat more whole grains, eggs, and leafy greens.

4. Probiotics

- **Why They Work**: A healthy gut microbiome influences how your body handles stress. Probiotics can reduce cortisol and improve mood.
- **Sources**: Choose high-quality probiotic capsules or eat fermented foods like yogurt, kimchi, and sauerkraut.

Superfoods for Cortisol Control

Superfoods are nutrient-dense ingredients that can work wonders for stress relief. Here are some lesser-known options to consider:

1. Matcha
- **Why It Works**: Matcha contains L-theanine, an amino acid that promotes relaxation without drowsiness. It also offers a gentle energy boost.
- **How to Use It**: Whisk matcha powder into hot water or milk for a calming tea. It's also great in smoothies or baked goods.

2. Dark Berries
- **Why They Work**: Blueberries, blackberries, and raspberries are packed with antioxidants that reduce inflammation triggered by stress.
- **How to Use Them**: Toss into yogurt, oatmeal, or salads for a burst of color and flavor.

3. Turmeric
- **Why It Works**: Curcumin, the active compound in turmeric, fights inflammation and oxidative stress.
- **How to Use It**: Add turmeric to curries, soups, or golden milk. Pair it with black pepper to enhance absorption.

4. Pumpkin Seeds
- **Why They Work**: Rich in magnesium, zinc, and tryptophan, pumpkin seeds support relaxation and cortisol regulation.
- **How to Use Them**: Sprinkle over salads, blend into pesto, or snack on them raw.

5. Aloe Vera Juice
- **Why It Works**: Aloe vera helps reduce inflammation and supports digestion, both of which are critical during stress.
- **How to Use It**: Drink a small glass of pure aloe vera juice or mix it into smoothies.

Hydration: The Overlooked Hero

Dehydration can amplify cortisol levels and make stress feel worse. Staying properly hydrated is one of the simplest ways to support your body.

1. Infused Water

Add flavor and nutrients to your water with these combinations:

- **Cucumber and Mint**: Refreshing and cooling.
- **Lemon and Ginger**: Supports digestion and immunity.
- **Berries and Basil**: Rich in antioxidants.

2. Coconut Water

Coconut water is an excellent source of electrolytes, which help combat the effects of stress. Drink it on its own or use it as a base for smoothies.

Practical Tips for Integration

It's one thing to know about stress-busting ingredients, but making them a regular part of your routine is where the magic happens. Here are some actionable ways to incorporate these into your daily life:

1. **Start Small**: Begin by adding one new ingredient to your meals each week. For example, sprinkle chia seeds over your morning oatmeal or swap your usual tea for matcha.
2. **Pre-Plan Your Pantry**: Stock up on staples like turmeric, ashwagandha, nuts, and dark chocolate. Having these on hand makes it easier to create stress-relieving meals.
3. **Batch Prep Adaptogen Blends**: Mix adaptogen powders like ashwagandha and maca into a pre-made blend. Keep it in a jar and scoop it into smoothies or coffee as needed.
4. **Create Relaxing Rituals**: Pair calming drinks like chamomile tea or golden milk with evening relaxation routines. These small moments can have a big impact on stress levels.
5. **Experiment with Recipes**: Try stress-relief recipes like a turmeric-laced soup, a smoothie with dark berries and matcha, or roasted pumpkin seeds with a sprinkle of cinnamon.

Sample Meal Plan for Stress Relief

Here's a simple daily plan that incorporates these ideas:
- **Breakfast**: Matcha latte and oatmeal topped with pumpkin seeds, dark berries, and a drizzle of honey.
- **Snack**: Greek yogurt with a sprinkle of chia seeds and fresh blueberries.
- **Lunch**: Spinach and quinoa salad with grilled salmon, avocado, and a turmeric dressing.
- **Snack**: A handful of almonds and a cup of tulsi tea.
- **Dinner**: Lentil curry spiced with turmeric and ginger, served with a side of steamed broccoli.
- **Evening Drink**: Warm golden milk with ashwagandha.

Stress is a part of life, but it doesn't have to take over. By adding adaptogens, supplements, superfoods, and hydration strategies to your routine, you'll equip your body to handle stress more effectively. Think of these nutritional hacks as tools in your wellness toolbox—always there to support you when life feels overwhelming.

Part 3: Lifestyle Reset – The Mind-Body Connection

CHAPTER 7

Sleep Smarter, Not Longer

Sleep is more than just a way to recharge; it's a cornerstone of health. When it comes to cortisol, your body's stress hormone, sleep plays a significant role in keeping it balanced. Poor sleep can send cortisol levels soaring, creating a cycle of stress and fatigue that feels impossible to escape. The good news is that with a few adjustments, you can improve your sleep quality and give your body the reset it needs.

How Sleep Impacts Cortisol Regulation

Cortisol follows a natural rhythm, peaking in the morning to help you wake up and gradually declining throughout the day. This cycle is known as the cortisol awakening response. Sleep disturbances, however, can throw this rhythm out of sync.

When you don't sleep well:

1. **Cortisol Spikes**: Poor sleep increases cortisol production, making you feel wired and tired simultaneously.
2. **Delayed Recovery**: Your body uses deep sleep to repair and recover. Without it, stress lingers in your system longer.
3. **Disrupted Hormones**: Sleep loss affects other hormones like melatonin (sleep regulator) and insulin (blood sugar regulator), compounding the problem.

Common Sleep Disruptors

To improve sleep, it helps to identify what's standing in the way. Here are some of the most common disruptors:

1. Blue Light Exposure

Screens from phones, tablets, and TVs emit blue light, which interferes with melatonin production. This makes it harder to fall asleep.

2. Erratic Schedules

Irregular bedtimes confuse your body's internal clock, making it harder to establish a consistent sleep rhythm.

3. Stress and Overthinking

A racing mind can make falling asleep feel impossible. Stress triggers cortisol, keeping your brain on high alert when it should be winding down.

4. Late-Night Caffeine or Alcohol

Both caffeine and alcohol can disrupt your natural sleep patterns. While caffeine is a stimulant, alcohol reduces deep sleep, leaving you feeling unrefreshed.

5. Environment

Noise, light, or even an uncomfortable mattress can prevent you from entering deep sleep.

Practical Tips for Better Sleep

Improving your sleep doesn't have to be complicated. Here are actionable steps to support restful nights and balanced cortisol:

1. Limit Screen Time Before Bed

- **Why**: Avoid screens at least an hour before bed to reduce blue light exposure.
- **How**: Switch to reading a physical book or listening to calming music instead of scrolling through your phone.

2. Stick to a Sleep Schedule

- **Why**: Going to bed and waking up at the same time every day helps regulate your body's clock.
- **How**: Choose a realistic bedtime and stick to it, even on weekends.

3. Create a Relaxing Bedtime Routine
- **Why**: A calming routine signals to your brain that it's time to wind down.
- **How**: Incorporate activities like gentle stretching, journaling, or sipping herbal tea.

4. Adjust Your Diet
- **Why**: Heavy meals, caffeine, and sugar close to bedtime can interfere with sleep.
- **How**: Opt for light, sleep-friendly snacks like a banana with almond butter or a small handful of walnuts.

5. Make Your Bedroom a Sleep Sanctuary
- **Why**: Your environment affects your ability to relax.
- **How**: Keep your bedroom cool, dark, and quiet. Invest in blackout curtains and a comfortable mattress.

<u>Creating the Perfect Nighttime Routine</u>

A nighttime routine is like a bridge between your day and sleep. Here's an example of a stress-relieving routine that promotes deeper rest:

1. Wind Down (60 Minutes Before Bed)
- **Dim the Lights**: Reduce the brightness in your home to signal your body that it's time to relax.
- **Unplug**: Turn off screens and switch to offline activities like reading or meditating.

2. Prepare Your Body (30 Minutes Before Bed)
- **Stretch or Do Yoga**: Gentle movements can release tension and calm your nervous system. Try a few simple stretches like forward bends or child's pose.
- **Sip Herbal Tea**: Chamomile, lavender, or valerian tea can promote relaxation and sleepiness.

3. Prepare Your Space (15 Minutes Before Bed)
- **Set the Temperature**: Aim for a cool room (around 65°F or 18°C).
- **Declutter**: A clean, organized bedroom feels more inviting and restful.

- **Use Aromatherapy**: Lavender essential oil can help you relax and fall asleep faster.

4. Sleep Affirmations (Just Before Bed)
- **Quiet the Mind**: Repeat calming affirmations or practice deep breathing. For example, inhale for four counts, hold for seven, and exhale for eight.

Foods That Promote Restful Sleep

Incorporate these into your diet to naturally support better sleep and cortisol balance:

1. **Bananas**: High in magnesium and potassium, which relax muscles.
2. **Almonds**: Provide magnesium, a mineral linked to better sleep.
3. **Kiwi**: Contains serotonin, which converts to melatonin.
4. **Tart Cherries**: A natural source of melatonin.
5. **Oats**: Contain nutrients that promote serotonin production.

Pair these foods with calming teas like chamomile or passionflower for an extra sleep boost.

Hydration and Sleep

Dehydration can cause discomfort, leading to restless nights. Here's how to stay hydrated without disrupting your sleep:
- **Drink Water Throughout the Day**: Aim for steady hydration rather than chugging large amounts in the evening.
- **Limit Fluids Before Bed**: Avoid drinking large amounts of water an hour before bedtime to reduce nighttime bathroom trips.

The Connection Between Exercise and Sleep

Physical activity can improve sleep quality, but timing matters:
- **Morning or Afternoon Exercise**: Boosts daytime energy and promotes better sleep at night.

- **Evening Exercise**: Avoid intense workouts close to bedtime, as they can raise cortisol levels and delay sleep.

Instead, opt for calming activities like yoga or a leisurely walk in the evening.

Early Warning Signs of Sleep Deprivation

Sometimes, poor sleep creeps up on you. Here's how to recognize the signs:
- **Daytime Fatigue**: Struggling to stay awake or alert during the day.
- **Irritability**: Feeling more emotional or reactive than usual.
- **Cravings**: Reaching for sugary or carb-heavy snacks to boost energy.
- **Brain Fog**: Difficulty concentrating or remembering details.

If any of these sound familiar, it's time to reassess your sleep habits.

Sleep is a powerful tool for managing cortisol and overall health. By understanding the relationship between sleep and stress, addressing common disruptors, and creating supportive habits, you can take control of your nights and wake up feeling refreshed.

Think of this process as an investment in yourself. Small changes—like swapping your evening screen time for a calming book or adding a lavender diffuser to your bedroom—can make a huge difference. With consistency, these habits become second nature, leading to better rest and a more balanced life.

CHAPTER 8

STRESS MANAGEMENT THAT STICKS

Managing stress is a skill, and like any skill, it can be learned and honed with the right tools and techniques. When stress takes over, cortisol levels rise, which can lead to fatigue, irritability, and a range of long-term health issues. Fortunately, there are effective ways to keep stress in check, tailored for different lifestyles. This chapter offers actionable, science-backed strategies to make stress management a lasting part of your life.

The Science Behind Stress Relief

Cortisol is your body's primary stress hormone, released in response to challenges or perceived threats. While short-term spikes in cortisol can be beneficial—helping you react quickly to danger—chronic stress keeps this hormone elevated, wreaking havoc on your body.

Stress management techniques, such as mindfulness, breathing exercises, and gentle movement, help activate the parasympathetic nervous system, also known as the "rest and digest" mode. This counteracts cortisol and promotes relaxation, balance, and healing.

Stress-Relief Techniques for Every Lifestyle

No two lives are the same. A strategy that works for a busy parent may not fit the schedule of an office worker or a student. Below, we'll explore universal techniques that can be adapted to fit your unique lifestyle.

1. Breathing Exercises: Quick Calm at Your Fingertips

Your breath is one of the most accessible tools for stress relief. Deep breathing sends a message to your brain that it's safe to relax.

- **The Science**: Controlled breathing reduces heart rate, lowers blood pressure, and decreases cortisol levels.
- **Try This: Box Breathing**
    1. Inhale through your nose for 4 seconds.
    2. Hold your breath for 4 seconds.
    3. Exhale slowly through your mouth for 4 seconds.

4. Hold again for 4 seconds.

Repeat this cycle for 1-2 minutes whenever you feel overwhelmed.

- **Lifestyle Fit**: Perfect for busy parents between tasks, office workers during a coffee break, or students before an exam.

2. Mindfulness Practices: Be Present, Feel Grounded

Mindfulness is the practice of being fully present in the moment, without judgment.

- **The Science**: Studies show that mindfulness reduces cortisol, improves emotional regulation, and increases resilience to stress.
- **How to Start**:
  - Begin with a 5-minute mindfulness meditation. Sit comfortably, close your eyes, and focus on your breath. Notice the sensation of air entering and leaving your nostrils.
  - For those on the go, try a mindful walk: focus on the rhythm of your steps, the feel of the ground beneath you, and the sounds around you.
- **Lifestyle Fit**: Can be practiced during a commute, while cooking, or even during a work break.

3. Gratitude Journaling: Shift Your Perspective

Gratitude journaling shifts your focus from what's wrong to what's right in your life.

- **The Science**: Regular gratitude practice has been linked to lower cortisol levels and increased happiness.
- **How to Do It**: Each evening, write down three things you're grateful for. Be specific—for example, "I'm grateful for the sunny weather during my lunch break today."
- **Lifestyle Fit**: A five-minute habit that's easy to incorporate into a nighttime routine, no matter how busy you are.

4. Gentle Movement: Exercise That Heals, Not Hurts

When it comes to stress relief, not all exercise is created equal. High-intensity workouts can sometimes elevate cortisol further, especially if your body is already under stress. Gentle, restorative movement is a better choice for managing cortisol.

- **The Science**: Activities like yoga, tai chi, and walking activate the parasympathetic nervous system, promoting relaxation while still providing physical benefits.
- **Exercise Ideas**:
    - **Yoga**: Focus on slow, deep stretches and controlled breathing.
    - **Tai Chi**: A meditative practice combining flowing movements with mindfulness.
    - **Walking**: A 20-minute stroll in nature can significantly lower cortisol levels.
- **Lifestyle Fit**: These activities are low-impact and can be done almost anywhere, making them accessible for all ages and fitness levels.

5. Progressive Muscle Relaxation: Release Tension

Stress often manifests as physical tension. Progressive muscle relaxation helps you identify and release this tension.

- **The Science**: This technique reduces cortisol by teaching your body to relax consciously.
- **How to Do It**:
    1. Start at your feet and work your way up.
    2. Tense each muscle group for 5 seconds, then release completely.
    3. Notice the difference between tension and relaxation.
- **Lifestyle Fit**: A calming activity to do before bed or during a stressful moment.

Stress-Busting Superfoods

Your diet has a direct impact on your stress levels. Certain foods can help regulate cortisol and support your body's response to stress.

Top Superfoods for Stress Relief

1. **Avocado**: Packed with healthy fats and potassium, avocados help lower blood pressure.
2. **Dark Chocolate**: Contains magnesium and compounds that reduce cortisol.
3. **Salmon**: Rich in omega-3 fatty acids, which combat inflammation caused by stress.
4. **Berries**: High in antioxidants that protect your body from the effects of chronic stress.
5. **Chamomile Tea**: Known for its calming properties and ability to lower cortisol.
6. **Spinach**: Full of magnesium, which helps relax muscles and reduce anxiety.
7. **Almonds**: Provide a mix of B vitamins and magnesium to support stress management.

Incorporating Stress-Relief Techniques into Daily Life

Here's how you can blend these techniques into your routine, no matter how packed your schedule is:

For Busy Parents
- Start your morning with a 5-minute breathing exercise before the kids wake up.
- Take mindful moments while doing everyday tasks like folding laundry or washing dishes.

For Office Workers
- Do box breathing during a coffee break.
- Take a walk around the office or step outside for fresh air.

For Students

- Use progressive muscle relaxation before studying to reduce tension.
- Practice gratitude journaling to shift your focus from stress to positivity.

Sample Stress-Relief Routine

Here's a simple, adaptable routine you can try:

Morning
- 5 minutes of gratitude journaling.
- A light breakfast with stress-busting foods like avocado on whole-grain toast.

Midday
- A 20-minute walk during lunch.
- Practice mindful eating by focusing on flavors, textures, and aromas.

Evening
- Unplug from screens an hour before bed.
- Sip chamomile tea while practicing progressive muscle relaxation.

Building Habits That Stick

Consistency is key. Start small by choosing one or two techniques from this chapter and integrating them into your life. As these habits become second nature, add more strategies.

Stress management isn't about eliminating stress completely—it's about equipping yourself with tools to handle it effectively. With practice, these techniques can help you feel calmer, more focused, and in control, no matter what life throws your way.

CHAPTER 9

Building a Low-Stress Environment

Stress doesn't just come from deadlines or major life events. Often, it's the accumulation of daily irritants, like a cluttered workspace, overwhelming digital notifications, or strained relationships, that take a toll. Crafting a low-stress environment—both physically and mentally—can make a significant difference in how you feel and function every day.

This chapter focuses on practical steps to simplify your space, balance your relationships, and address the silent stressors of modern life, like technology.

Decluttering for Calm: The Power of Simplicity

A cluttered space can lead to a cluttered mind. Research shows that visual chaos increases cortisol levels, making it harder to relax or concentrate. Creating order in your surroundings helps foster a sense of calm and control.

Start with Your Physical Space

- **Clear the Essentials First**: Focus on the areas you use most, like your bedroom, kitchen, or workspace. A clear desk or a made bed can set the tone for a less stressful day.
- **The "One Year Rule"**: If you haven't used something in the past year, consider donating or discarding it. Holding onto unused items can subconsciously weigh you down.
- **Divide and Conquer**: Decluttering can feel overwhelming, so tackle one small section at a time. For example, start with a single drawer rather than an entire room.

Mental Decluttering

Just like physical clutter, mental clutter—worrying, overthinking, or holding onto unresolved issues—can increase stress.

- **Try Brain-Dumping**: At the end of the day, write down everything on your mind. Seeing your thoughts on paper can help you sort and prioritize them.
- **Set Boundaries on Multitasking**: Focus on one task at a time. Multitasking often leads to mistakes and mental fatigue, which add to stress.

- **Adopt a Gratitude Practice**: Spending even five minutes listing things you're grateful for can reframe your mindset and reduce mental clutter.

Technology: The Hidden Stressor

Modern technology is a double-edged sword. While it keeps us connected and productive, constant notifications, emails, and social media can overstimulate your mind and spike cortisol.

Digital Detox Strategies

- **Audit Your Apps**: Delete apps that don't add value to your life. Keep only those that are essential or genuinely helpful.
- **Set Notification Boundaries**: Turn off non-essential alerts. For emails, consider setting specific times of day to check them instead of responding as they arrive.
- **Create Screen-Free Zones**: Dedicate certain areas of your home—like the bedroom or dining table—as screen-free zones to encourage relaxation and presence.

Using Technology Mindfully

While it's important to set limits, technology can also be a tool for stress relief when used intentionally.
- **Meditation Apps**: Apps like Calm or Headspace guide you through stress-relieving exercises.
- **Smart Lighting**: Some smart bulbs mimic natural light, helping you feel more relaxed in the evenings and energized during the day.
- **Soothing Soundscapes**: Play calming music or nature sounds to create a tranquil environment.

Building Stress-Free Relationships

Your relationships play a significant role in either alleviating or amplifying stress. Toxic dynamics, unspoken frustrations, or lack of boundaries can lead to emotional strain.

Nurturing Healthy Connections

- **Practice Active Listening**: Make an effort to really hear the other person without interrupting or planning your response while they're speaking. This fosters better understanding and reduces misunderstandings.
- **Communicate Clearly**: Be honest about your feelings, but approach difficult conversations with kindness and empathy. Saying "I feel overwhelmed when…" instead of "You always…" keeps the focus on your experience rather than blaming the other person.
- **Invest Time in Positive Relationships**: Make time for people who uplift and support you. Even short interactions with friends or loved ones can significantly reduce stress.

Setting Boundaries

Boundaries aren't about shutting people out—they're about protecting your energy.

- **Learn to Say No**: It's okay to decline invitations or requests if they feel overwhelming. A simple, "I can't take that on right now, but thank you for thinking of me," works well.
- **Limit Toxic Interactions**: If certain relationships consistently drain you, minimize contact or find ways to keep interactions brief and neutral.

Managing Stress at Work

For many, work is a primary source of stress. Balancing responsibilities while maintaining well-being requires thoughtful strategies.

Creating a Calming Workspace

- **Personalize Your Desk**: Add calming elements, like a small plant, a photo of a loved one, or a soothing scent diffuser.
- **Organize Regularly**: A clutter-free workspace can improve focus and reduce the overwhelm that comes from searching for misplaced items.
- **Invest in Comfort**: Ergonomic chairs, keyboards, and even wrist supports can make your workspace more inviting and reduce physical strain.

Prioritize and Delegate

- **Use the "3 D's" Rule**: When faced with a task, decide whether to Do, Delegate, or Delete it.
- **Focus on the Big Picture**: Start each day by identifying your top three priorities. Completing meaningful work first can reduce the stress of minor distractions later.

Take Micro-Breaks

Short breaks can refresh your mind and body. Stand up, stretch, or take a quick walk to reset. Even stepping away for 5 minutes can improve focus and lower stress.

Creating a Low-Stress Home Environment

Your home should feel like a sanctuary—a place where you can relax and recharge.

Incorporate Calming Elements

- **Natural Light**: Open blinds during the day to let in sunlight. Natural light boosts mood and reduces fatigue.
- **Comfortable Textures**: Soft blankets, fluffy pillows, or a cozy rug can make a space feel more inviting.
- **Aromatherapy**: Scents like lavender, chamomile, or eucalyptus can help you unwind.

Establish Routines That Work for You

- **Morning Ritual**: Start your day with something calming, like stretching, journaling, or enjoying a quiet cup of tea.
- **Evening Wind-Down**: Dedicate time to transition from work mode to relaxation. This could include reading, a warm bath, or meditation.

Crafting a low-stress environment isn't about perfection—it's about creating a space and lifestyle that supports your well-being. Whether it's decluttering your home, setting boundaries with technology and relationships, or personalizing your workspace, each step you take can make a significant difference.

Choose one area to focus on this week. Maybe it's organizing your pantry, silencing non-essential notifications, or having an honest conversation with a loved one. Small changes can lead to big improvements in how you feel day-to-day.

Your environment should be a source of calm, not chaos. With intentional effort, you can create a space and routine that work for you—and your stress levels will thank you for it.

Part 4: The Cortisol Detox Diet Plan

CHAPTER 10

YOUR 20-DAY RESET PLAN

Embarking on a wellness journey can feel daunting, but a structured plan simplifies the process and keeps you focused. This 20-day reset plan is designed to help you jumpstart fat loss, balance your hormones, and build habits that support long-term health. It's straightforward, flexible, and ideal for beginners who want results without overcomplicating their routines.

This plan includes daily meals, practical grocery tips, and meal prep strategies to make life easier. Think of it as your guide to starting fresh, with motivation sprinkled throughout to keep you on track.

Plan Overview

How the Plan Works

- **Daily Structure**: Each day features three main meals and one optional snack.
- **Balanced Meals**: Every meal combines protein, healthy fats, and fiber-rich carbohydrates to stabilize blood sugar and support hormone health.
- **Flexible Options**: Swap ingredients based on preferences or availability while sticking to the nutritional framework.

Key Guidelines

- **Hydration**: Drink at least eight 8-ounce glasses of water daily. Add a splash of lemon or cucumber for flavor.
- **Mindful Eating**: Eat slowly and stop when you're satisfied, not stuffed.
- **Prep in Advance**: Set aside time each week to prepare ingredients or batch-cook meals to save time during busy days.

20-Day Reset Plan Table

DAY	BREAKFAST	LUNCH	DINNER	SNACKS(OPTIONAL)
1	Greek yogurt with fresh berries and a drizzle of honey	Grilled chicken salad with avocado and olive oil dressing	Baked salmon with roasted asparagus and quinoa	Handful of almonds with an apple
2	Scrambled eggs with spinach and tomatoes	Turkey wrap with hummus and mixed greens	Beef stir-fry with broccoli and cauliflower rice	Carrot sticks with guacamole
3	Chia pudding with almond milk, vanilla, and sliced banana	Quinoa bowl with roasted veggies and chickpeas	Herb-roasted chicken with sweet potatoes and green beans	Hard-boiled egg with cucumber slices
4	Smoothie: spinach, frozen mango, protein powder, and almond milk	Tuna salad on mixed greens with olive oil and lemon	Grilled shrimp with zucchini noodles and marinara	Greek yogurt with a handful of walnuts
5	Oatmeal topped with almond butter and fresh raspberries	Leftover grilled chicken with steamed broccoli and olive oil	Pork tenderloin with roasted Brussels sprouts and wild rice	Handful of mixed seeds

6	Avocado toast on whole-grain bread with a poached egg	Lentil soup with a side of mixed greens	Baked cod with roasted carrots and mashed cauliflower	Celery sticks with almond butter
7	Smoothie: kale, frozen pineapple, chia seeds, and coconut water	Grilled chicken Caesar salad (light dressing)	Beef meatballs with spaghetti squash and marinara	Handful of dark chocolate chips
8	Omelet with mushrooms, onions, and a slice of whole-grain toast	Turkey burger (lettuce wrap) with sweet potato fries	Lemon-garlic shrimp with sautéed spinach and quinoa	Sliced pear with almond butter
9	Overnight oats with chia seeds, almond milk, and strawberries	Chicken and veggie stir-fry with brown rice	Grilled salmon with avocado salsa and roasted zucchini	Handful of roasted chickpeas
10	Cottage cheese with sliced peaches and a sprinkle of cinnamon	Greek quinoa salad with cucumber, olives, and feta	Herb-crusted pork chop with sautéed kale and mashed sweet potato	Baby carrots with tahini dip

11	Smoothie: spinach, banana, protein powder, and unsweetened almond milk	Grilled shrimp salad with mango and cilantro dressing	Grilled chicken with roasted Brussels sprouts and wild rice	Small handful of cashews
12	Scrambled eggs with avocado slices and whole-grain toast	Lentil and veggie curry over cauliflower rice	Baked salmon with roasted sweet potatoes and steamed broccoli	Sliced cucumber with tzatziki
13	Greek yogurt with granola and fresh blueberries	Turkey wrap with guacamole and spinach	Beef chili with a side of roasted green beans	Handful of sunflower seeds
14	Smoothie bowl with frozen berries, spinach, almond milk, and granola	Grilled chicken Caesar wrap (light dressing)	Garlic shrimp with zucchini noodles and pesto	Greek yogurt with chia seeds
15	Chia pudding with sliced mango and coconut flakes	Chicken and veggie stir-fry with quinoa	Herb-roasted turkey breast with mashed cauliflower and green beans	Small piece of dark chocolate
16	Omelet with	Lentil and	Baked cod	Handful of

	diced bell peppers and a side of mixed greens	spinach soup with whole-grain bread	with lemon butter sauce and steamed asparagus	roasted almonds
17	Oatmeal with sliced almonds and fresh blackberries	Mediterranean salad with chickpeas, cucumber, and tahini dressing	Pork loin with roasted carrots and quinoa	Apple slices with peanut butter
18	Smoothie: kale, frozen mango, chia seeds, and unsweetened coconut milk	Grilled shrimp salad with avocado and lime dressing	Chicken stir-fry with broccoli and cauliflower rice	Handful of trail mix
19	Cottage cheese with sliced kiwi and a drizzle of honey	Grilled turkey burger (lettuce wrap) with roasted sweet potato fries	Garlic-roasted salmon with sautéed spinach and brown rice	Hard-boiled egg with cherry tomatoes
20	Greek yogurt parfait with granola and fresh raspberries	Quinoa and roasted veggie bowl with tahini drizzle	Grilled chicken breast with roasted Brussels sprouts and mashed sweet potatoes	Sliced cucumber with hummus

Grocery Shopping Tips

1. **Stick to a List**
   Plan your meals for the week and make a detailed shopping list. Sticking to it helps avoid impulse purchases and ensures you have all the ingredients needed.

2. **Shop the Perimeter**
   Focus on the outer sections of the store where fresh produce, proteins, and dairy are located. Limit time in processed food aisles.

3. **Choose Versatile Ingredients**
   Pick items that can be used in multiple meals, like spinach (for smoothies, salads, or omelets) and sweet potatoes (as a side, in bowls, or mashed).

4. **Buy in Bulk**
   Stock up on pantry staples like quinoa, lentils, nuts, and olive oil. These items have a long shelf life and can save money in the long run.

5. **Prioritize Fresh Over Packaged**
   Opt for fresh vegetables, fruits, and proteins. When buying packaged items, check for minimal ingredients and no added sugars.

Meal Prep Strategies

1. **Batch Cook Proteins**
   Prepare proteins like grilled chicken, baked salmon, or turkey meatballs in bulk. Store them in airtight containers for easy use throughout the week.

2. **Prep Veggies in Advance**
   Wash, chop, and portion vegetables ahead of time. Store them in the fridge for quick access when making stir-fries, salads, or side dishes.

3. **Portion Out Snacks**
   Divide snacks like nuts, seeds, or chopped fruits into individual portions. This prevents overeating and makes healthy choices more convenient.

4. **Use Freezer-Friendly Recipes**
   Cook double portions of meals like soups or chili and freeze half for later. This saves time and reduces food waste.

5. **Label and Organize**
   Clearly label containers with the meal name and date. This ensures nothing gets forgotten or wasted.

Motivational Words to Keep You Committed

You've got this! Starting something new always takes a bit of effort, but each day brings you closer to your goal. Treat this 20-day reset as an investment in yourself—a chance to feel more energized, balanced, and confident. Remember, progress is progress, no matter how small. Celebrate every win, whether it's trying a new recipe, sticking to your plan, or simply feeling better in your body.

Think of this reset not as a diet but as a way to nourish yourself inside and out. Small steps lead to big results, so take it one meal, one grocery trip, and one day at a time. Your health and happiness are worth it!

Gr ocery Shopping List for 20-Day Reset Plan

Here's a detailed shopping list organized by category to help you prepare for the 20-day reset plan. This list covers everything you'll need for the meals and snacks throughout the plan.

CATEGORY	Item	Quantity/Amount
Proteins	Chicken breast	6-8 breasts
	Ground turkey	2 lbs
	Salmon fillets	4 fillets
	Shrimp	1 lb
	Pork tenderloin	2 lbs
	Eggs	2 dozen
	Tuna (canned, packed in water)	2 cans

	Greek yogurt	32 oz
	Cottage cheese	16 oz
Vegetables	Spinach	2 large bags
	Kale	1 bunch
	Sweet potatoes	5-6 medium-sized
	Zucchini	4 medium
	Broccoli	2 heads
	Asparagus	1 bunch
	Green beans	1 lb
	Bell peppers (red, yellow,	3-4 peppers

green)	
Carrots	1 lb
Cucumber	2 medium
Tomatoes (Roma or cherry)	1 pint
Brussels sprouts	1 lb
Cauliflower (for rice or mashed)	1 large head
Mushrooms	1 package
Avocados	5-6 medium
Fruits	
Bananas	5-6 medium

	Berries (blueberries, raspberries)	2-3 cups
	Apples	4-6 medium
	Peaches	2-3 medium
	Mango	2 large
	Pineapple (fresh or frozen)	1 small
	Pears	3-4 medium
	Kiwi	3-4 medium
Grains and Starches	Quinoa	1 lb
	Brown rice	1 lb

	Whole-grain bread	1 loaf
	Oats (rolled or steel-cut)	1 lb
	Spaghetti squash	2 medium
Legumes & Nuts	Lentils (dry or canned)	1 lb dry or 2 cans
	Chickpeas (canned or dry)	2 cans or 1 lb dry
	Almonds	1 bag
	Cashews	1 bag
	Walnuts	1 bag
	Sunflower seeds	1 bag

	Pumpkin seeds	1 bag
Dairy & Alternatives	Almond milk	2-3 cartons
	Coconut milk (unsweetened)	1 can
Herbs & Spices	Garlic	1 bulb
	Ginger	1 small piece
	Fresh parsley	1 bunch
	Fresh cilantro	1 bunch
	Basil	1 bunch
	Cinnamon	1 jar
	Black pepper	1 jar

	Sea salt or Himalayan salt	1 jar
	Ground turmeric	1 jar
	Red pepper flakes	1 jar
	Chili powder	1 jar
	Cumin	1 jar
	Italian seasoning	1 jar
Oils & Vinegars	Olive oil	1 bottle
	Coconut oil	1 jar
	Apple cider vinegar	1 bottle

	Balsamic vinegar	1 bottle
Condiments & Sauces	Tahini	1 jar
	Mustard	1 jar
	Hummus	tub
	Low-sodium soy sauce	1 bottle
	Hot sauce	1 bottle
	Salsa	1 jar
Frozen	Frozen berries	1 bag
	Frozen spinach	1 bag
Snacks & Extras	Dark chocolate (70% cocoa or higher)	1 bar

Category	Item	Quantity
	Almond butter	1 jar
	Peanut butter	1 jar
	Granola (low-sugar)	1 bag
Beverages	Herbal teas (chamomile, peppermint)	1 box each
	Green tea	1 box
	Coffee (if desired)	1 bag

SHOPPING TIPS:

- **Fresh Produce**: Buy fruits and vegetables in quantities that align with the number of servings you'll need. If you can, purchase some frozen options like spinach and berries to ensure you always have them on hand without worrying about spoilage.
- **Protein Sources**: If possible, buy fresh protein and freeze it for future use. This helps prevent waste, especially if you're not planning to use it immediately.

- **Bulk Buying**: For pantry staples like quinoa, oats, and nuts, buying in bulk can save money and reduce packaging waste.
- **Seasonal**: Opt for seasonal produce whenever you can to ensure freshness and better prices.

By following this shopping list, you'll be equipped with everything you need to make your 20-day reset a success!

CHAPTER 11

RECIPES TO SUPPORT EVERY STAGE

Finding recipes that are quick and easy when you're busy, yet satisfying and nourishing when you have time to relax, can make a world of difference on your health journey. Whether you're starting your day, in the middle of a hectic afternoon, or winding down after a busy week, the right recipes can support your goals for fat loss, hormone balance, and overall wellness. In this chapter, we'll break down recipes into categories that fit various life scenarios—whether you need a "Quick Fix," a "Meal Prep Champion," or a comforting "Indulgent but Healthy" option for the weekend.

Quick Fixes (For Busy Mornings & Hectic Days)

When you're rushing through the morning or running from one task to the next, it's essential to have meals that are both fast and nourishing. These recipes are designed to fuel your day without taking up too much time or mental energy.

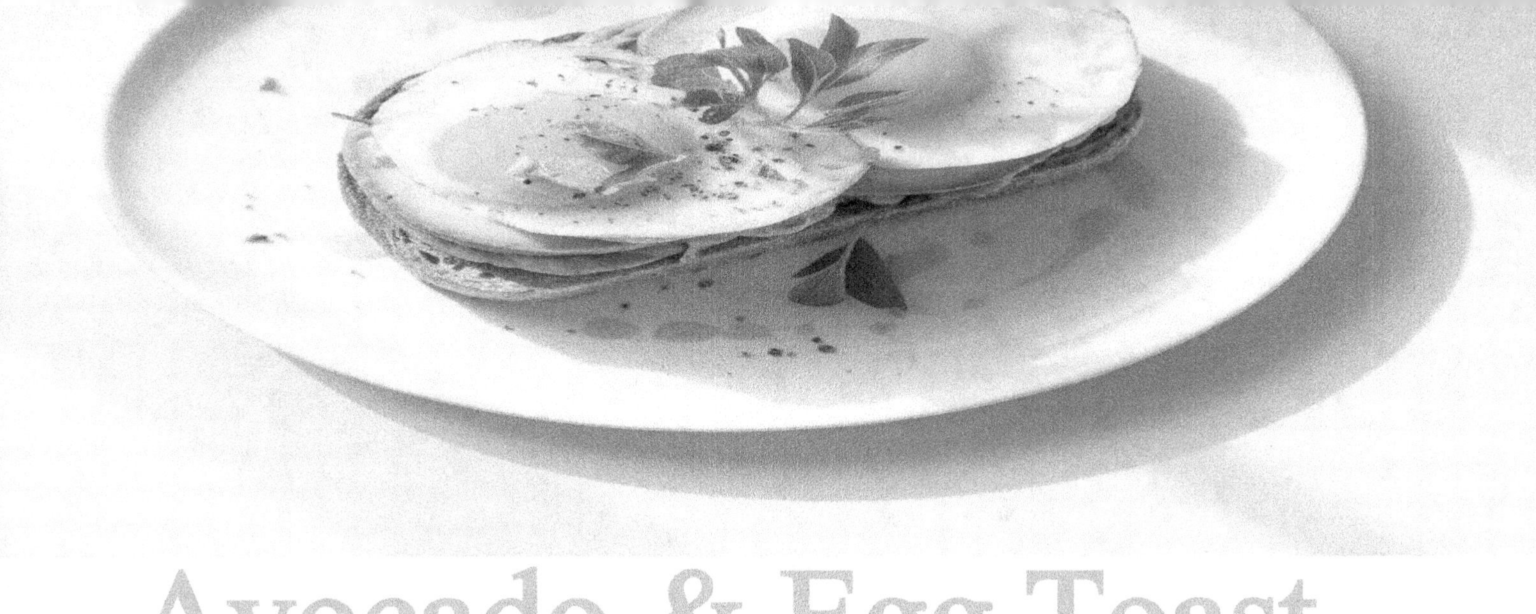

Avocado & Egg Toast

INGREDIENTS:

- 1 ripe avocado
- 1 slice whole-grain bread
- 2 eggs
- Sea salt and black pepper to taste
- Olive oil (for drizzling)

INSTRUCTIONS:

- Toast the bread to your liking.
- While the bread toasts, heat a little olive oil in a pan and cook the eggs to your preferred style (scrambled, fried, or poached).
- Mash the avocado and spread it generously on the toast.
- Top with eggs, season with salt and pepper, and drizzle with olive oil.

Prep time: 5 minutes
Cook time: 5 minutes

Nutritional Information:

- Calories: 350
- Protein: 14g
- Carbs: 30g
- Fats: 22g

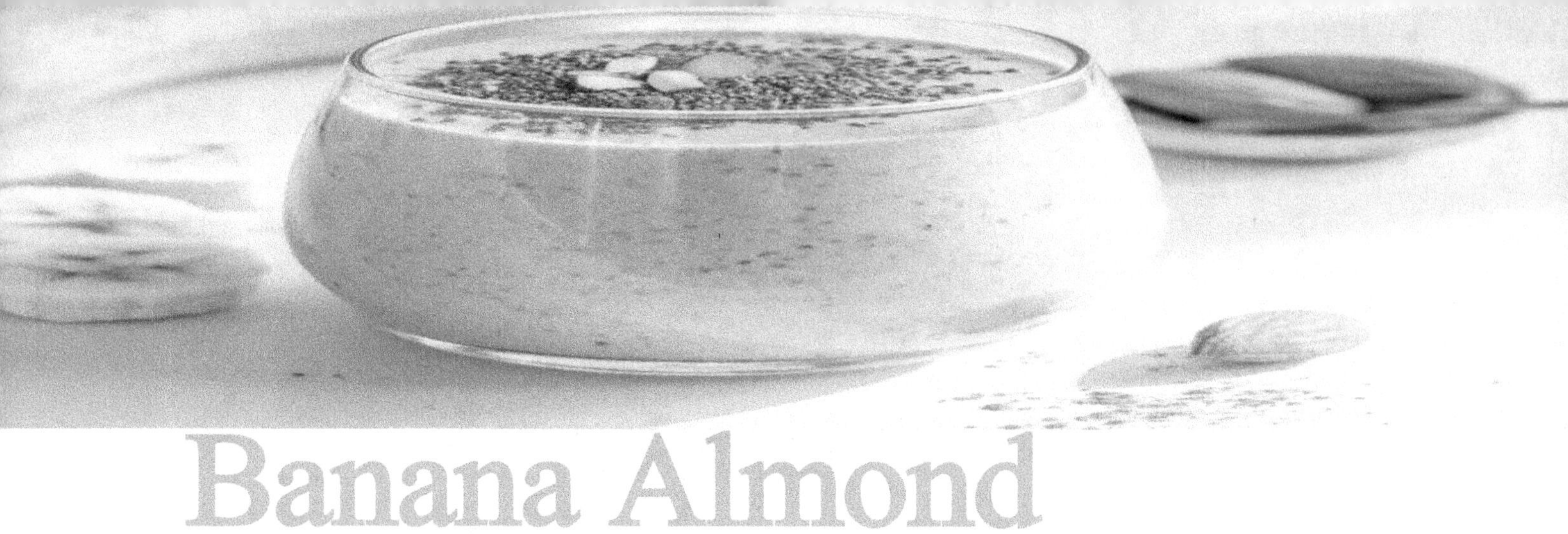

Banana Almond Smoothie

INGREDIENTS:

- 1 ripe banana
- 1 tbsp almond butter
- 1 cup almond milk
- 1 tbsp chia seeds
- 1 scoop protein powder (optional)

INSTRUCTIONS:

- Blend all ingredients in a high-speed blender until smooth.
- Pour into a glass and enjoy immediately.

Prep time: 3 minutes
Cook time: 0 minutes

Nutritional Information:

- Calories: 250
- Protein: 14g
- Carbs: 30g
- Fats: 12g

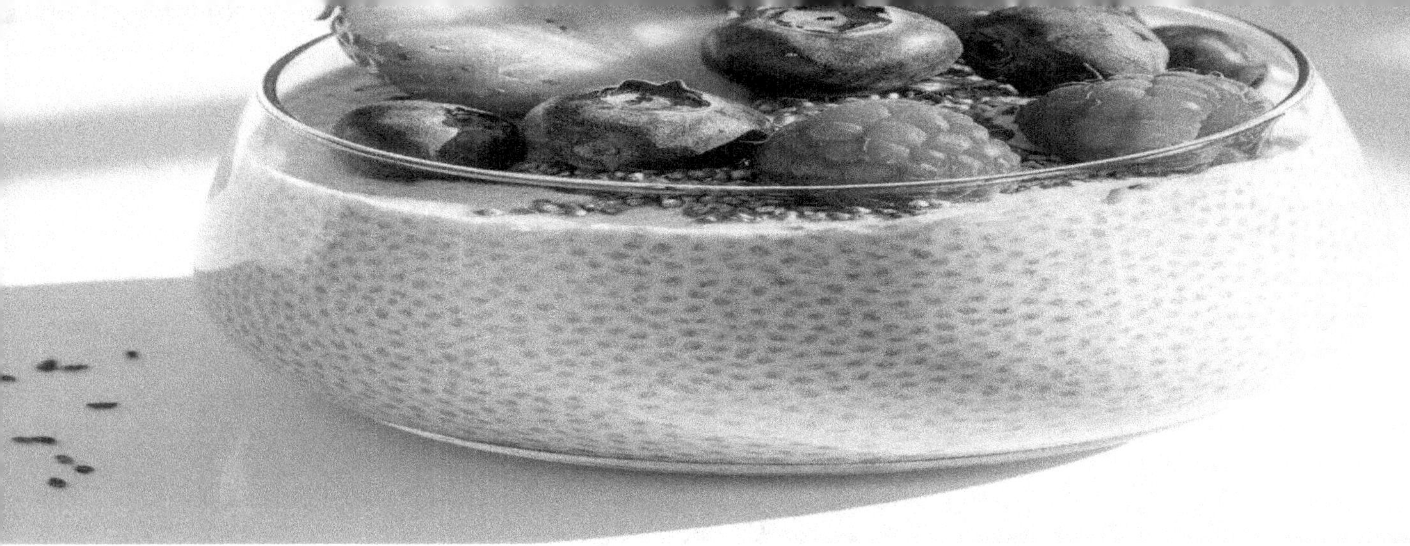

Chia Pudding with Berries

INGREDIENTS:
- 3 tbsp chia seeds
- 1 cup almond milk
- 1 tsp honey (optional)
- Fresh berries for topping

INSTRUCTIONS:
- Mix chia seeds, almond milk, and honey in a bowl or jar. Stir to combine.
- Let it sit in the fridge for at least 30 minutes or overnight.
- Top with fresh berries before serving.

Prep time: 3 minutes
Cook time: 0 minutes (refrigeration time varies)

Nutritional Information:
- Calories: 180
- Protein: 5g
- Carbs: 18g
- Fats: 12g

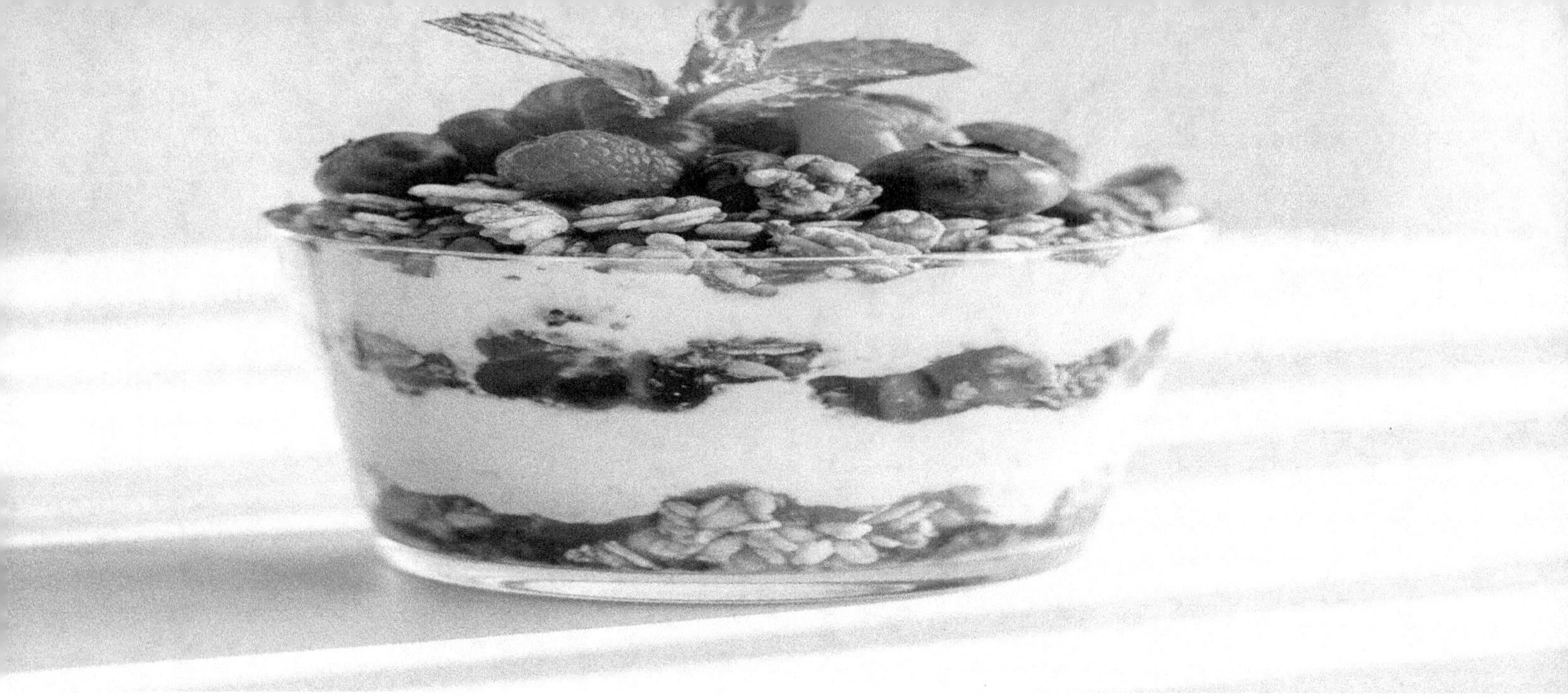

Greek Yogurt Parfait

INGREDIENTS:
- 1 cup Greek yogurt (unsweetened)
- 1/2 cup granola (low-sugar)
- 1/4 cup mixed berries

INSTRUCTIONS:
- Layer yogurt, granola, and berries in a bowl or jar.
- Serve immediately or store for later.

Prep time: 5 minutes
Cook time: 0 minutes

Nutritional Information:
- Calories: 220
- Protein: 15g
- Carbs: 24g
- Fats: 10g

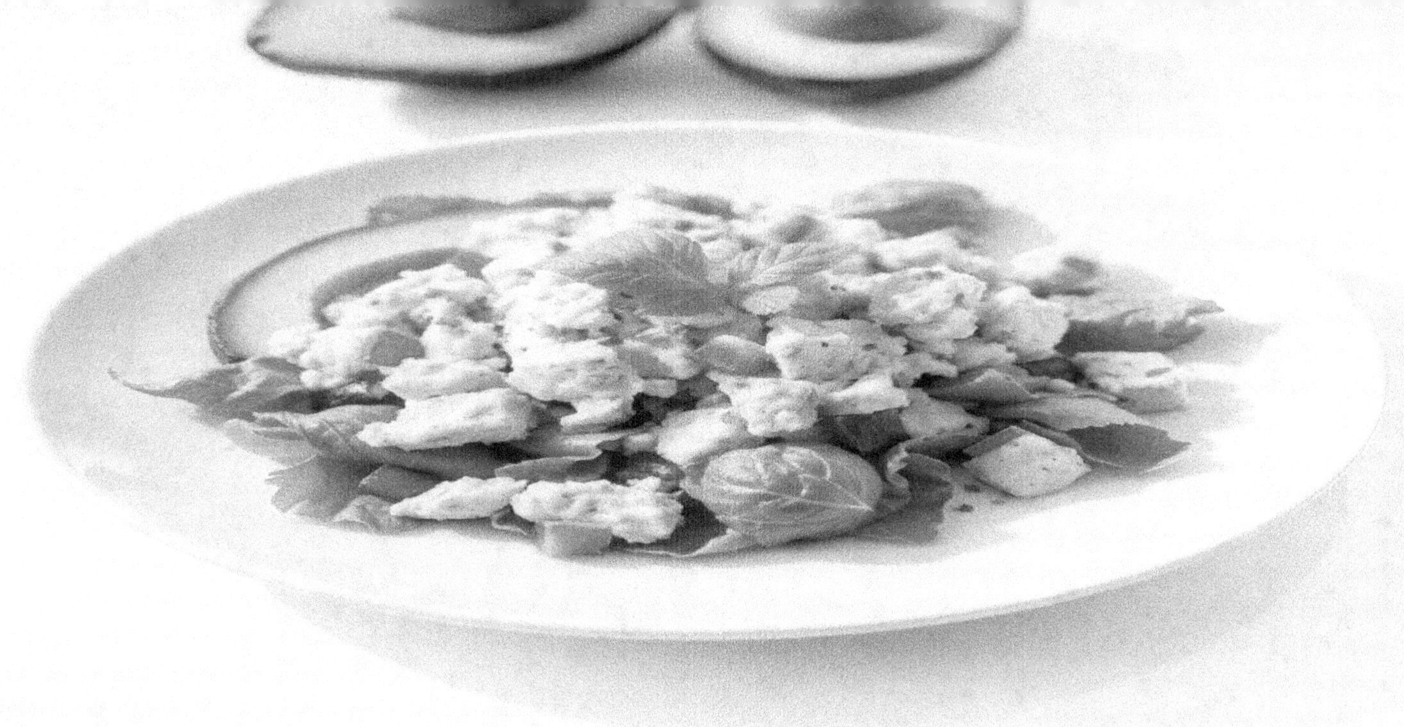

Avocado & Tuna Salad

INGREDIENTS:
- 1 avocado, diced
- 1 can tuna (packed in water), drained
- 1 tbsp olive oil
- 1 tsp lemon juice
- Salt and pepper to taste

INSTRUCTIONS:
- Mix all ingredients in a bowl.
- Serve as a salad or spread on whole-grain crackers.

Prep time: 5 minutes
Cook time: 0 minutes
Nutritional Information:
- Calories: 280
- Protein: 18g
- Carbs: 10g
- Fats: 20g

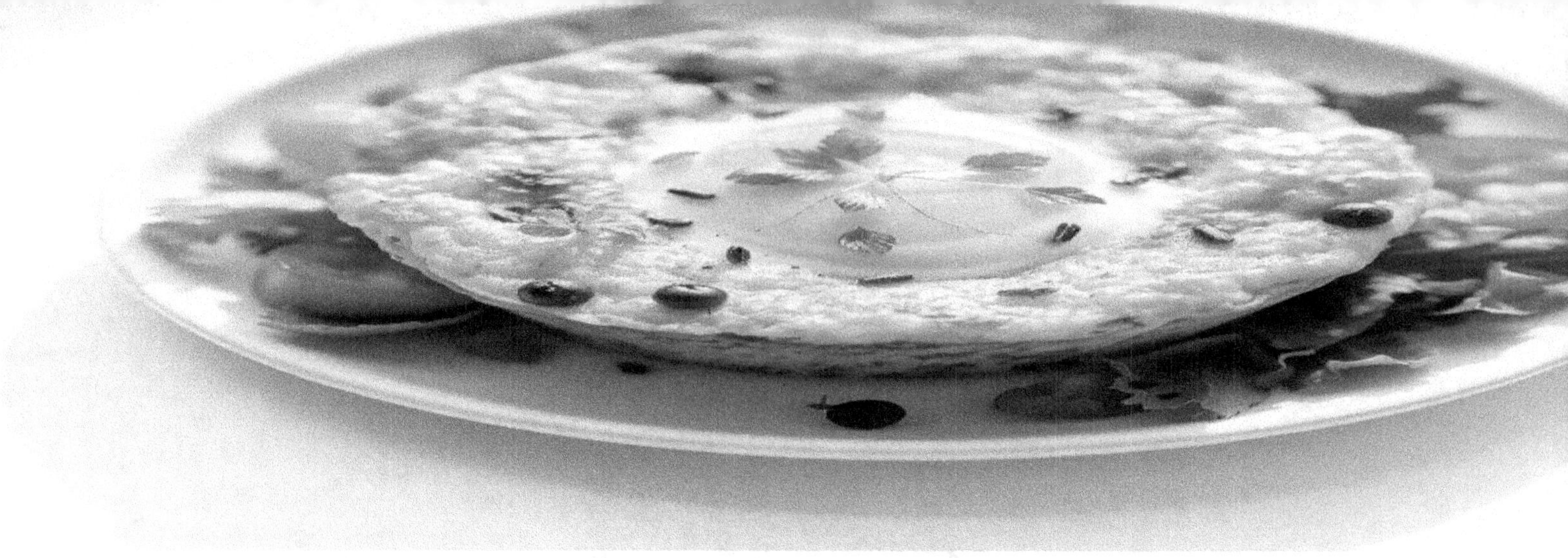

Veggie Egg Muffins

INGREDIENTS:
- 6 large eggs
- 1/2 cup chopped spinach
- 1/4 cup diced bell peppers
- 1/4 cup diced onion
- Salt and pepper to taste

INSTRUCTIONS:
- Preheat the oven to 350°F (175°C).
- Whisk the eggs and add vegetables, salt, and pepper.
- Pour into a muffin tin and bake for 20-25 minutes until set.
- Enjoy warm or store in the fridge for later.

Prep time: 10 minutes
Cook time: 20-25 minutes
Nutritional Information:
- Calories: 150
- Protein: 12g
- Carbs: 6g
- Fats: 10g

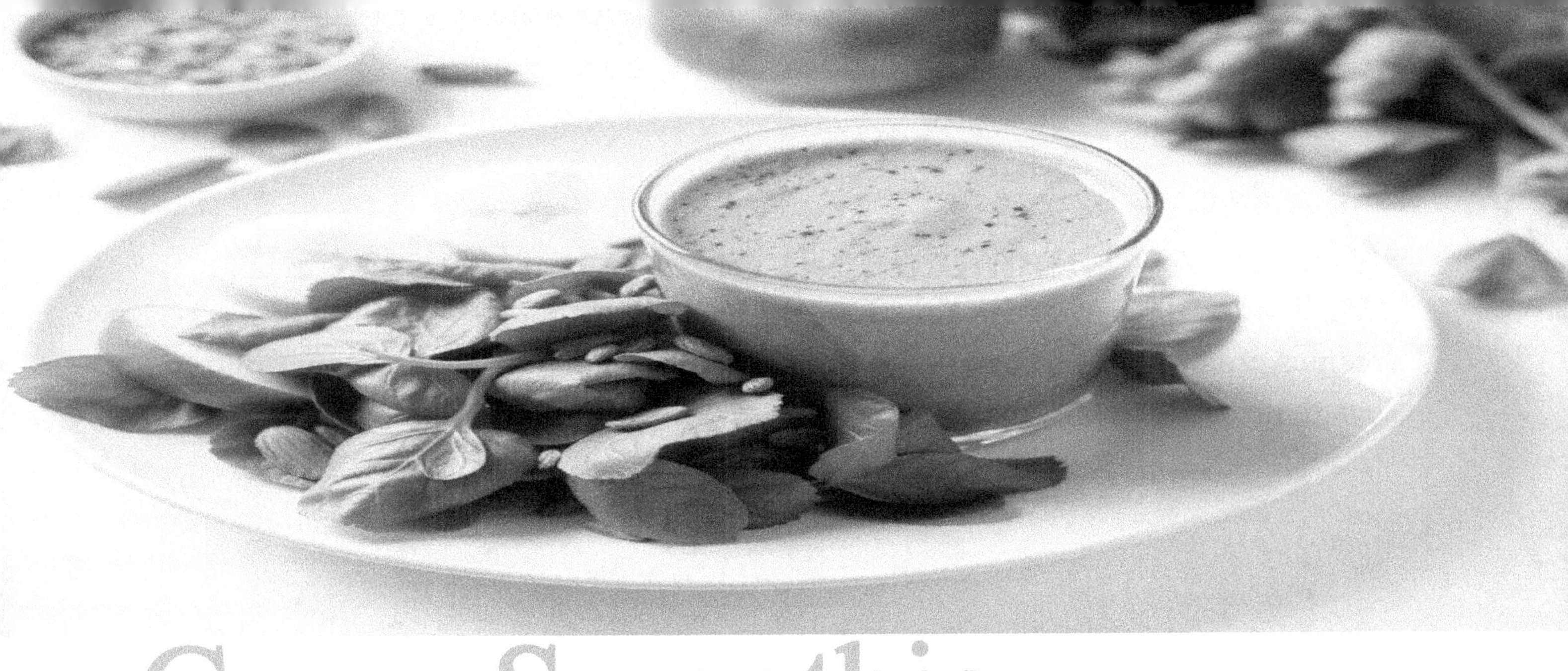

Green Smoothie

INGREDIENTS:

- 1 cup spinach
- 1/2 banana
- 1/2 apple
- 1 cup almond milk
- 1 tbsp flaxseeds

INSTRUCTIONS:

- Blend all ingredients in a blender until smooth.
- Enjoy as a refreshing, nutrient-packed start to your day.

Prep time: 5 minutes
Cook time: 0 minutes
Nutritional Information:

- Calories: 180
- Protein: 5g
- Carbs: 30g
- Fats: 6g

Meal Prep Champions (For Busy Weeks)

When you're preparing for a busy week, having meals ready to go is key. These recipes are designed to make meal prep easy and delicious while supporting your health goals.

Grilled Chicken with Roasted Vegetables

INGREDIENTS:
- 4 boneless, skinless chicken breasts
- 1 tbsp olive oil
- 1 tbsp Italian seasoning
- 2 cups mixed vegetables (zucchini, bell peppers, onions)

INSTRUCTIONS:
- Preheat the oven to 400°F (200°C).
- Toss vegetables with olive oil and seasoning, then spread on a baking sheet.
- Grill chicken breasts until fully cooked, about 6-7 minutes per side.
- Roast vegetables in the oven for 20-25 minutes.
- Serve chicken with roasted veggies.

Prep time: 10 minutes
Cook time: 30 minutes
Nutritional Information:
- Calories: 350
- Protein: 35g
- Carbs: 20g
- Fats: 18g

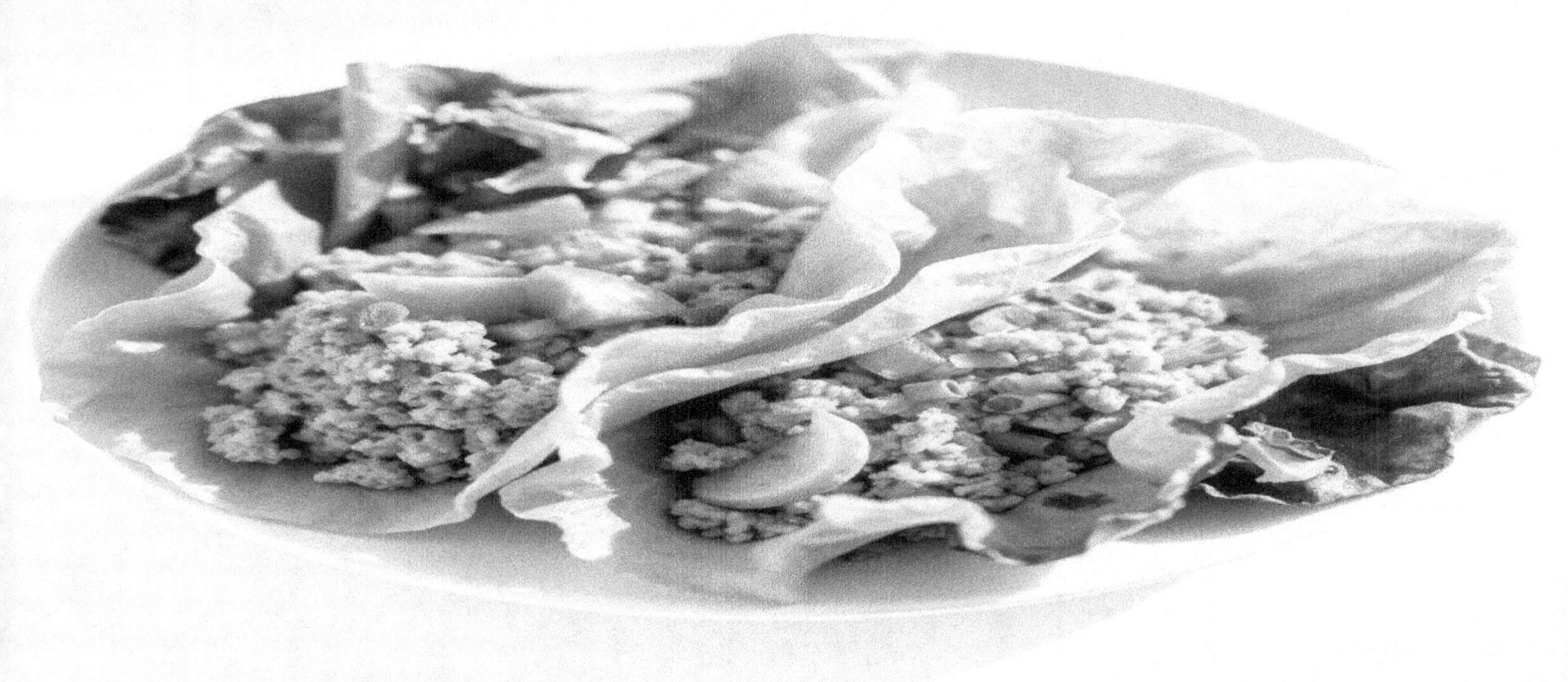

Turkey Lettuce Wraps

INGREDIENTS:

- 1 lb ground turkey
- 1 tbsp olive oil
- 1 tbsp soy sauce
- 1/2 cup chopped green onions
- Romaine lettuce leaves

INSTRUCTIONS:

- Cook turkey in olive oil over medium heat until browned.
- Stir in soy sauce and green onions, cooking for an additional 2-3 minutes.
- Spoon turkey mixture into lettuce leaves and serve.

Prep time: 10 minutes
Cook time: 10 minutes
Nutritional Information:

- Calories: 250
- Protein: 28g
- Carbs: 5g
- Fats: 14g

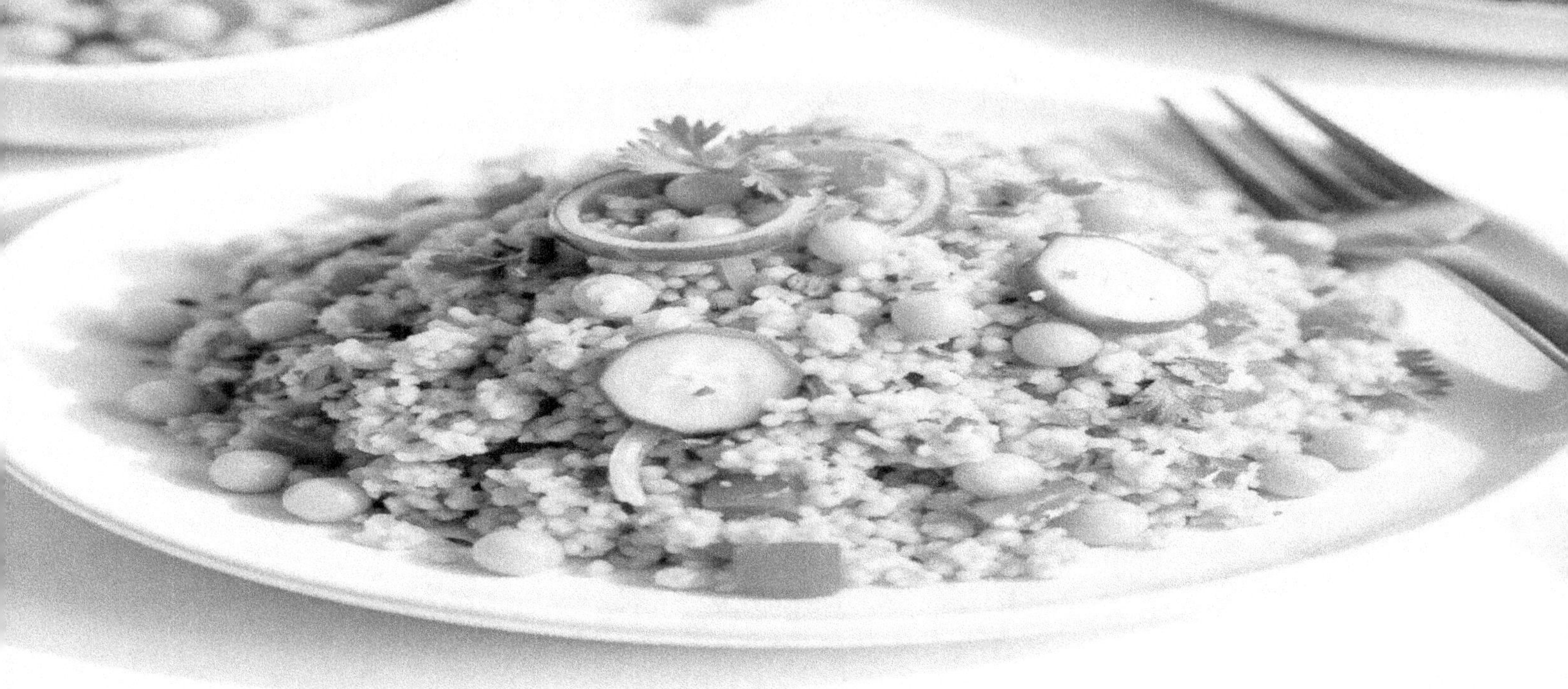

Quinoa & Chickpea Salad

INGREDIENTS:

- 1 cup cooked quinoa
- 1 can chickpeas (drained and rinsed)
- 1 cucumber, chopped
- 1/2 red onion, chopped
- Lemon vinaigrette dressing

INSTRUCTIONS:

- In a large bowl, combine quinoa, chickpeas, cucumber, and onion.
- Toss with lemon vinaigrette dressing.
- Store in the fridge for up to 3 days.

Prep time: 10 minutes

Cook time: 0 minutes

Nutritional Information:

- Calories: 300
- Protein: 10g
- Carbs: 45g
- Fats: 9g

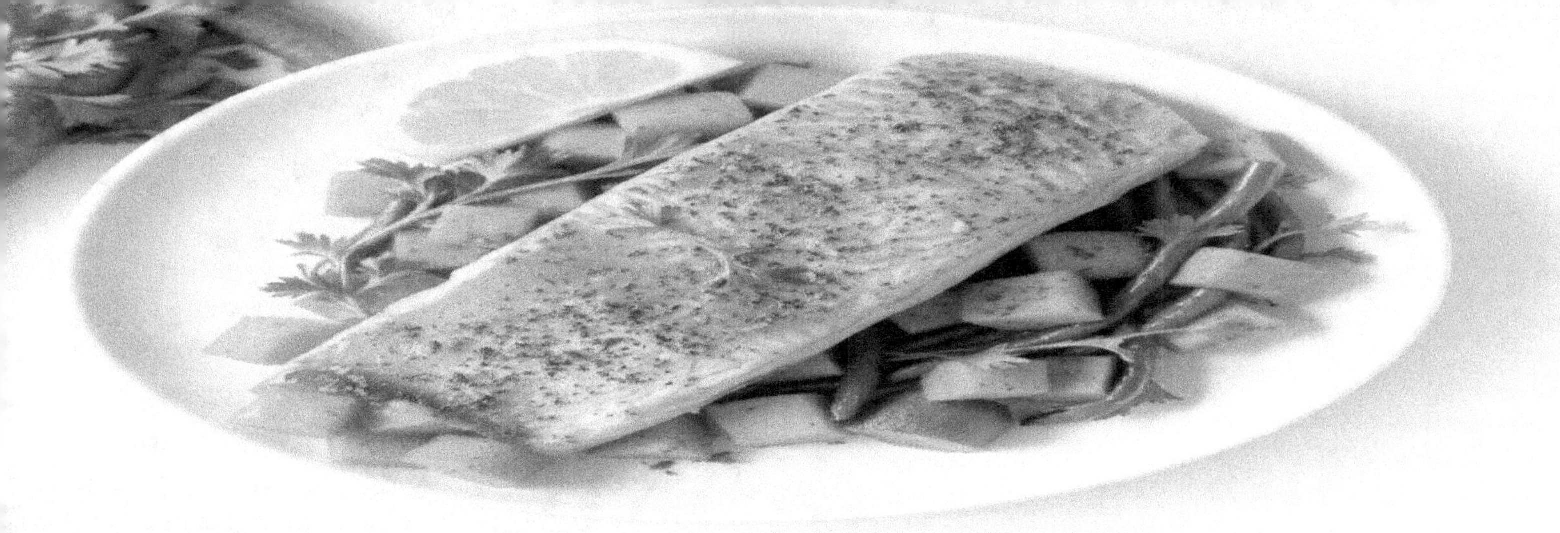

Baked Salmon with Sweet Potato

INGREDIENTS:

- 4 salmon fillets
- 2 sweet potatoes, diced
- 1 tbsp olive oil
- Salt and pepper to taste

INSTRUCTIONS:

- Preheat the oven to 400°F (200°C).
- Toss sweet potatoes with olive oil, salt, and pepper, then spread on a baking sheet.
- Bake for 25 minutes.
- Add salmon fillets to the sheet and bake for an additional 10-12 minutes.
- Serve together.

Prep time: 10 minutes

Cook time: 35 minutes

Nutritional Information:

- Calories: 450
- Protein: 35g
- Carbs: 40g
- Fats: 20g

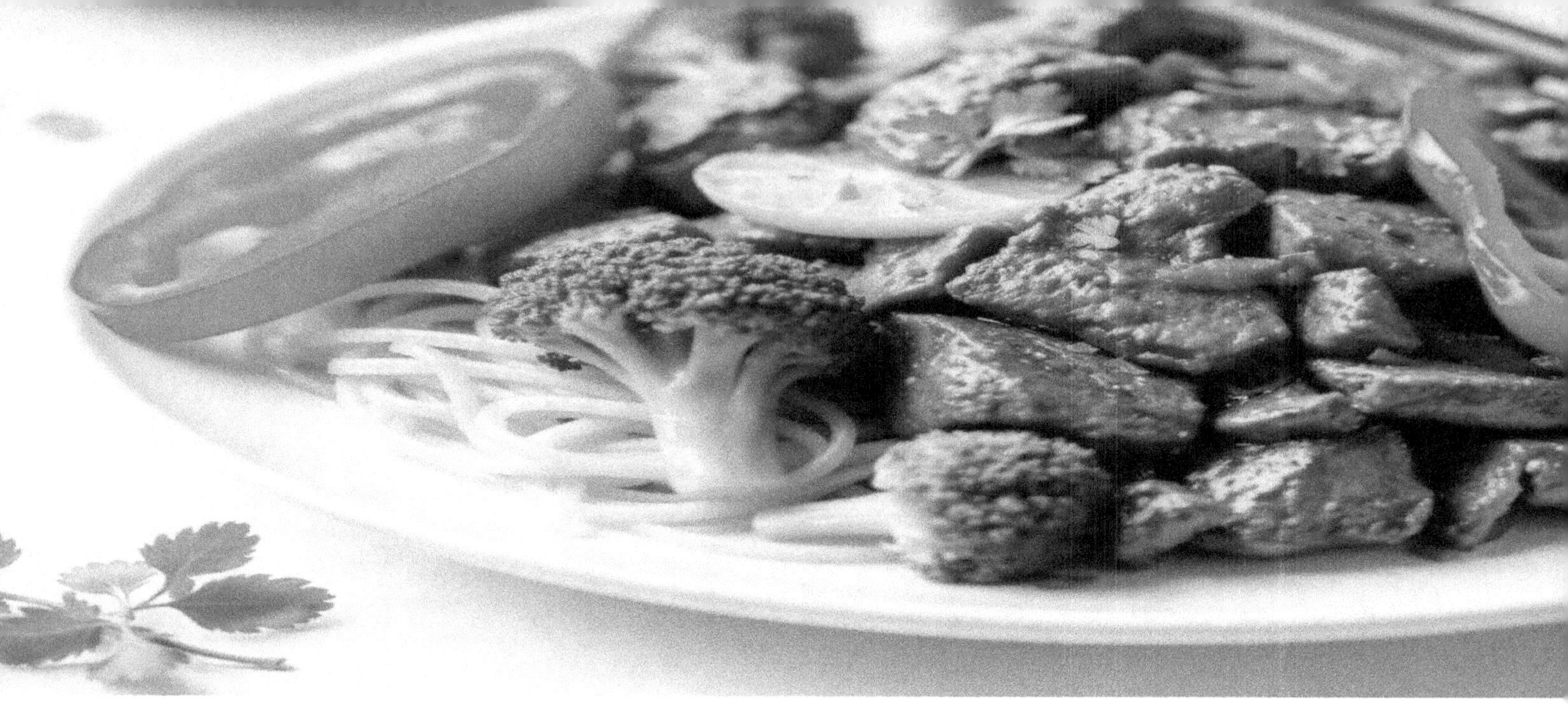

Beef Stir Fry

INGREDIENTS:

- 1 lb beef (sirloin or flank steak), thinly sliced
- 1 cup broccoli florets
- 1 red bell pepper, sliced
- 2 tbsp soy sauce
- 1 tbsp sesame oil

INSTRUCTIONS:

- Heat sesame oil in a pan over medium heat.
- Add beef and cook until browned.
- Add vegetables and soy sauce, and stir-fry for 5-7 minutes.
- Serve immediately or store for later.

Prep time: 10 minutes

Cook time: 10 minutes

Nutritional Information:

- Calories: 350
- Protein: 30g
- Carbs: 15g
- Fats: 20g

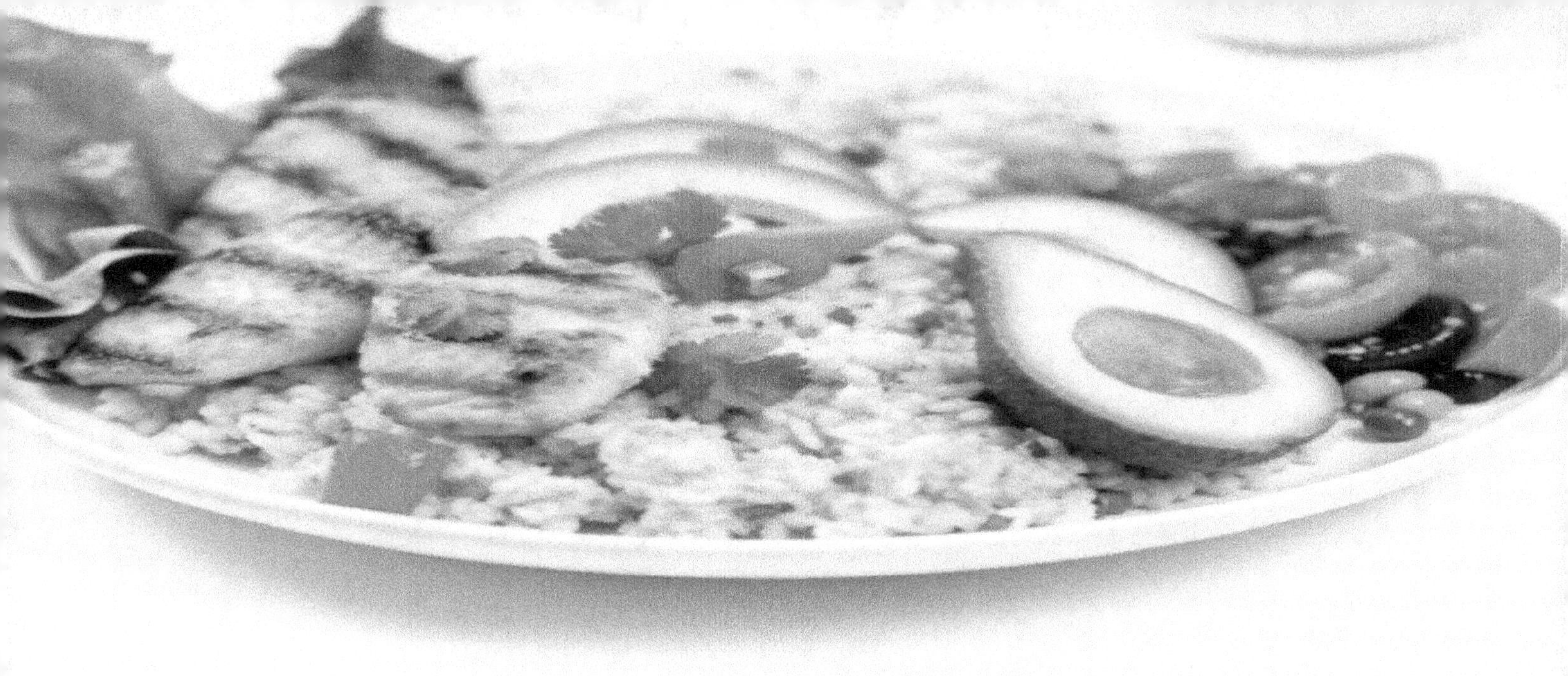

Chicken and Rice Bowls

INGREDIENTS:
- 4 chicken breasts, grilled
- 2 cups brown rice, cooked
- 1 avocado, sliced
- 1/2 cup salsa

INSTRUCTIONS:
- Layer rice, chicken, avocado, and salsa in bowls.
- Store in the fridge for an easy meal prep option.

Prep time: 5 minutes

Cook time: 30 minutes

Nutritional Information:
- Calories: 400
- Protein: 35g
- Carbs: 40g
- Fats: 15g

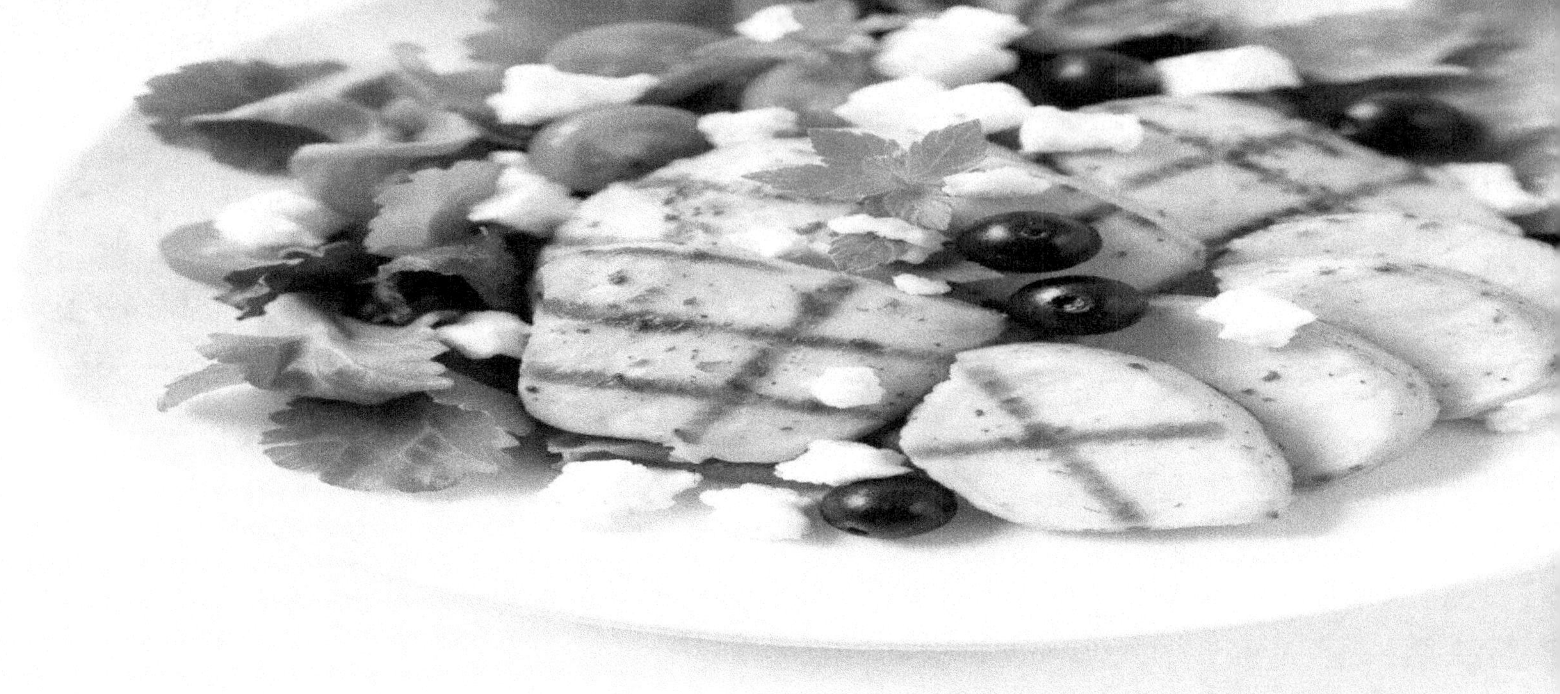

Mediterranean Chicken Salad

INGREDIENTS:

- 4 grilled chicken breasts, sliced
- 2 cups mixed greens
- 1/2 cup feta cheese
- 1/4 cup Kalamata olives
- 2 tbsp olive oil and vinegar dressing

INSTRUCTIONS:

- Toss mixed greens, chicken, feta, and olives in a bowl.
- Drizzle with dressing and serve.

Prep time: 5 minutes

Cook time: 0 minutes

Nutritional Information:

- Calories: 350
- Protein: 30g
- Carbs: 10g
- Fats: 20g

Indulgent but Healthy (Weekend Treats)

Weekends are the perfect time to enjoy something special without compromising your health goals. These recipes are both indulgent and nourishing, so you can satisfy cravings while staying on track.

Cauliflower Pizza Crust

INGREDIENTS:

- 1 head of cauliflower, grated
- 1 egg
- 1/2 cup mozzarella cheese
- 1 tsp oregano

INSTRUCTIONS:

- Preheat the oven to 400°F (200°C).
- Grate cauliflower and microwave it for 5 minutes. Let cool.
- Mix cauliflower, egg, cheese, and oregano.
- Spread on a baking sheet to form a crust.
- Bake for 20 minutes, then add your favorite toppings and bake for another 5-10 minutes.

Prep time: 10 minutes

Cook time: 25 minutes

Nutritional Information:

- Calories: 220
- Protein: 15g
- Carbs: 15g
- Fats: 15g

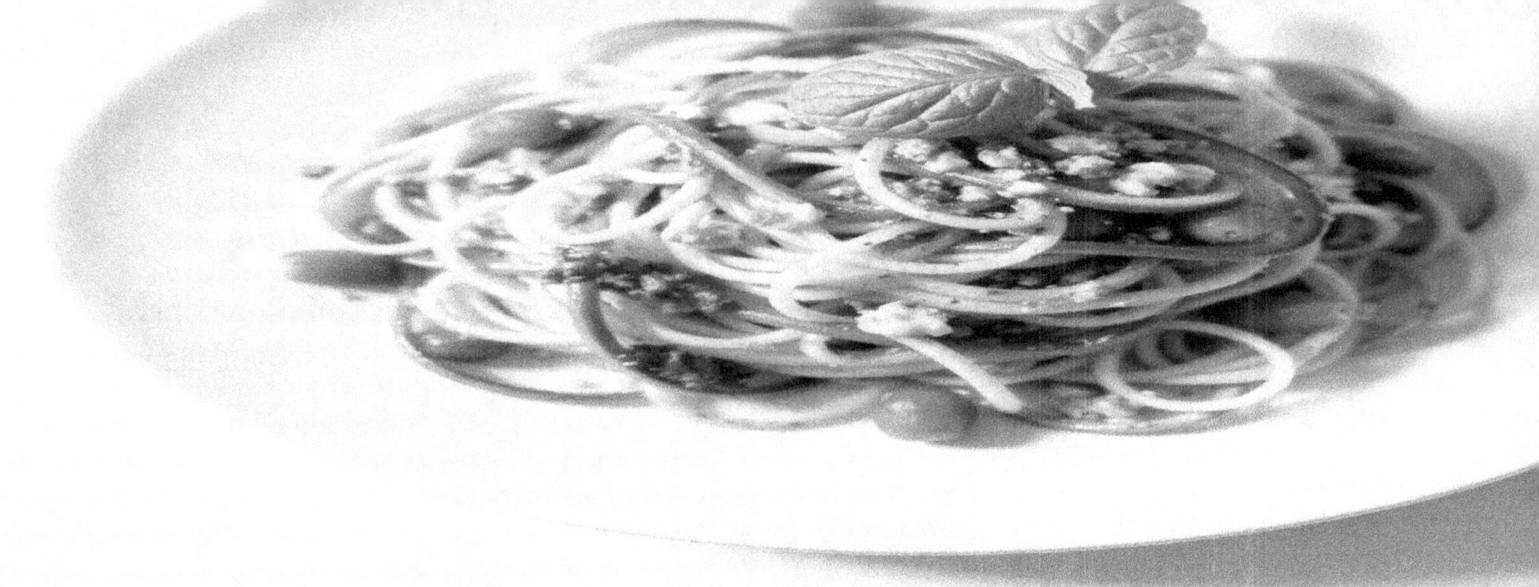

Zucchini Noodles with Pesto

INGREDIENTS:
- 2 zucchinis, spiralized
- 1/2 cup pesto
- 1 tbsp olive oil

INSTRUCTIONS:
- Sauté zucchini noodles in olive oil for 2-3 minutes.
- Toss with pesto and serve.

Prep time: 5 minutes
Cook time: 5 minutes

Nutritional Information:
Calories: 200
Protein: 5g
Carbs: 10g
Fats: 18g

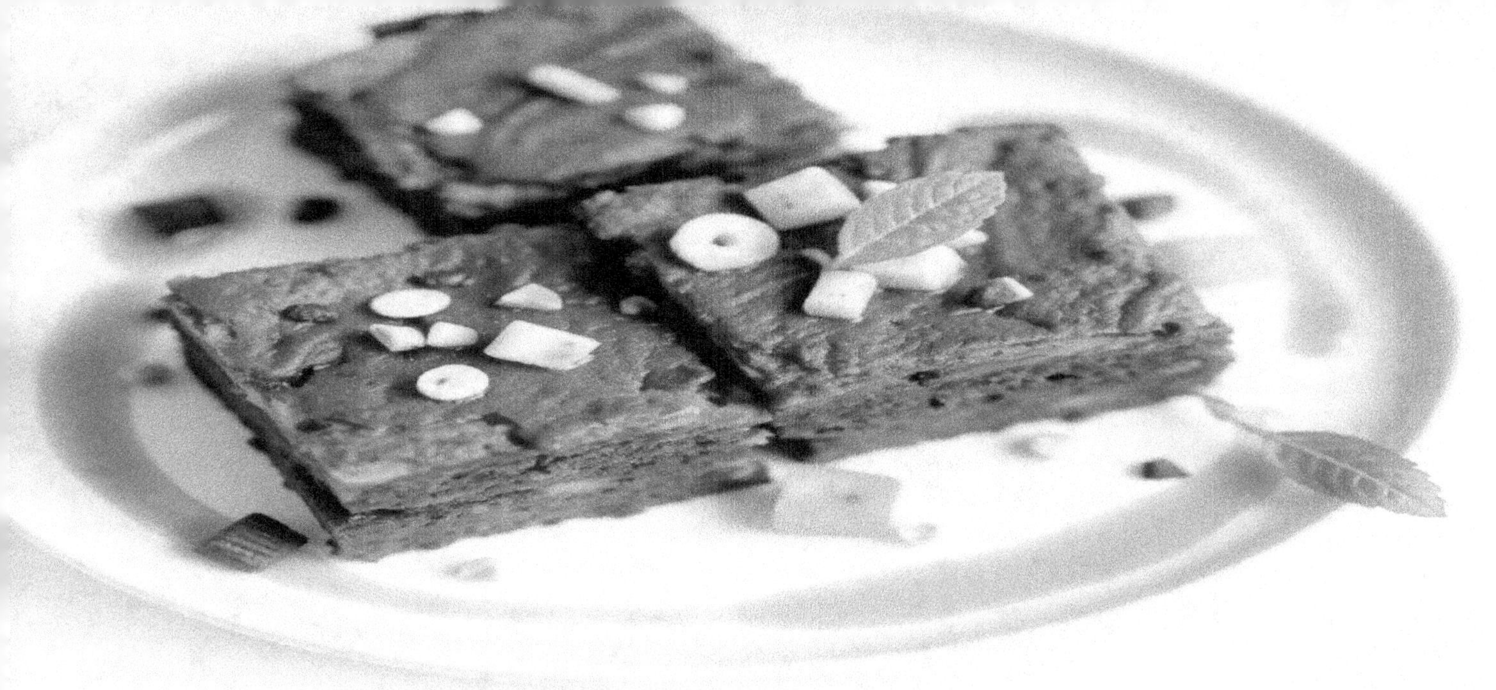

Sweet Potato Brownies

INGREDIENTS:
- 2 medium sweet potatoes, baked and mashed
- 1/2 cup almond flour
- 1/4 cup cocoa powder
- 2 eggs
- 1/4 cup maple syrup

INSTRUCTIONS:
- Preheat the oven to 350°F (175°C).
- Mix all ingredients in a bowl.
- Pour into a greased baking pan and bake for 20-25 minutes.

Prep time: 10 minutes
Cook time: 25 minutes
Nutritional Information:
- Calories: 180
- Protein: 4g
- Carbs: 25g
- Fats: 8g

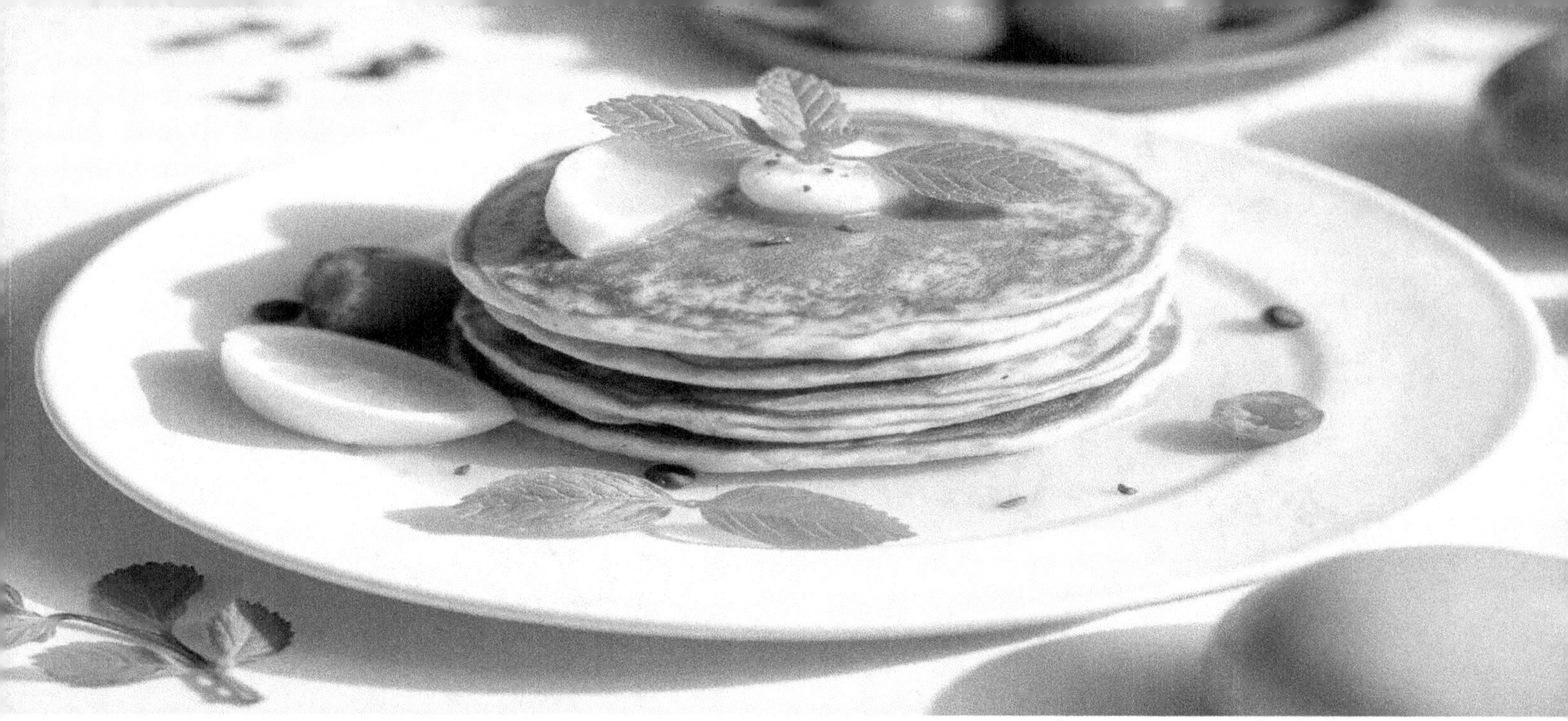

Paleo Pancakes

INGREDIENTS:

- 1 cup almond flour
- 2 eggs
- 1/4 cup almond milk
- 1 tsp vanilla extract

INSTRUCTIONS:

- Mix all ingredients into a smooth batter.
- Cook pancakes on a non-stick skillet over medium heat for 2-3 minutes per side.

Prep time: 5 minutes

Cook time: 10 minutes

Nutritional Information:

- Calories: 250
- Protein: 10g
- Carbs: 15g
- Fats: 18g

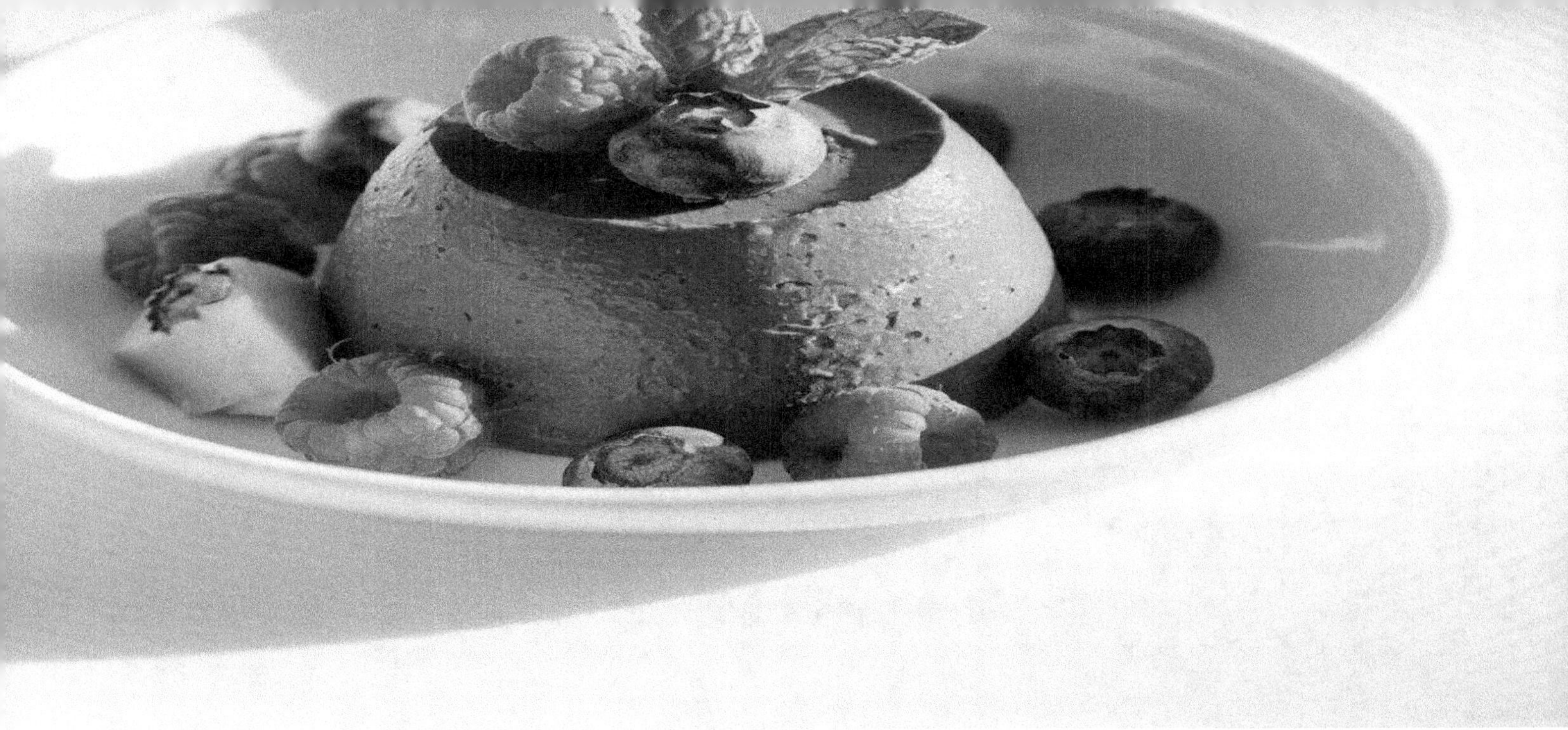

Dark Chocolate Avocado Mousse

INGREDIENTS:

- 1 ripe avocado
- 2 tbsp cocoa powder
- 1/4 cup maple syrup
- 1 tsp vanilla extract

INSTRUCTIONS:

- Blend all ingredients in a blender until smooth.
- Chill in the fridge for 30 minutes before serving.

Prep time: 5 minutes

Cook time: 0 minutes

Nutritional Information:

- Calories: 180
- Protein: 3g
- Carbs: 18g
- Fats: 12g

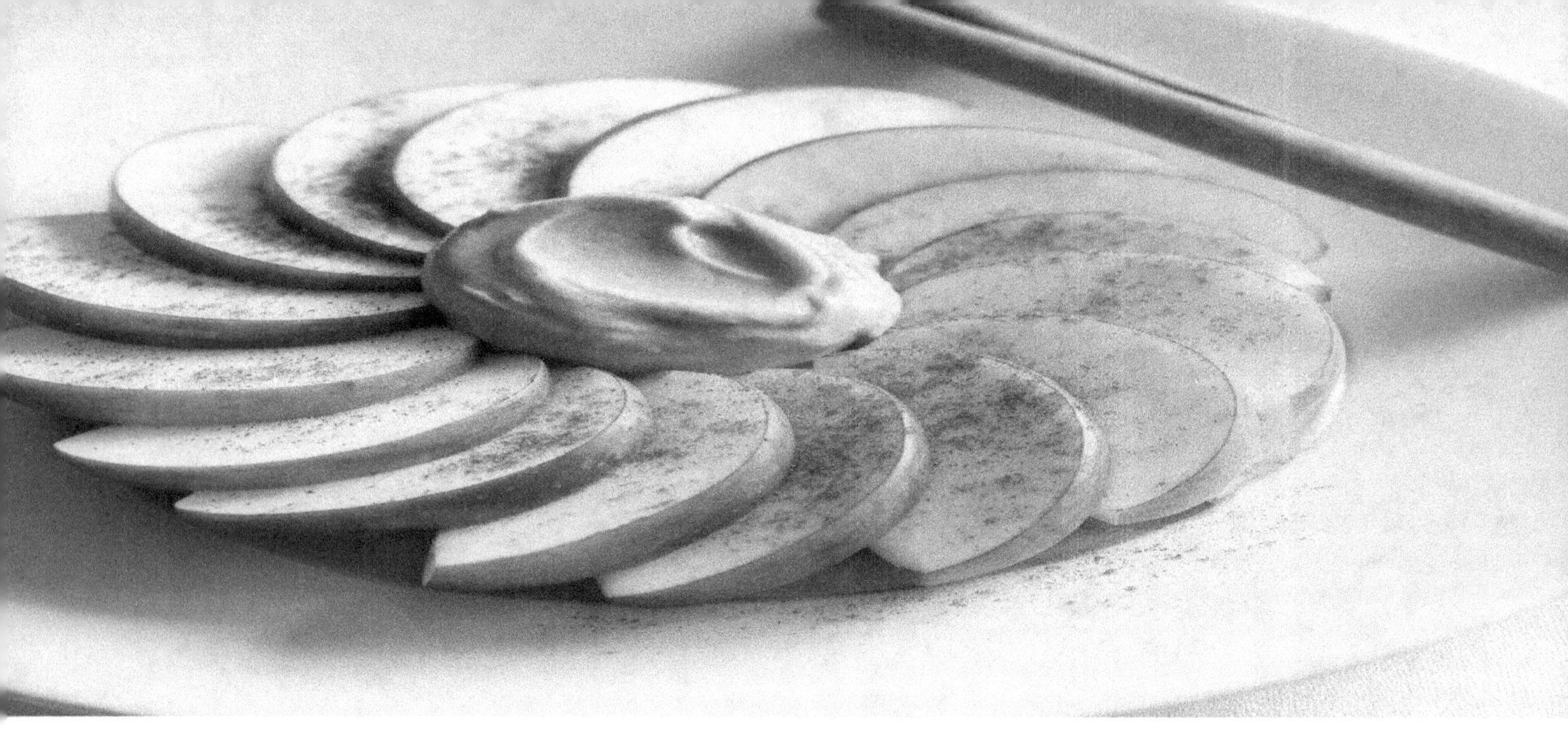

Baked Apple with Cinnamon

INGREDIENTS:

- 4 apples, cored
- 2 tbsp almond butter
- 1 tsp cinnamon

INSTRUCTIONS:

- Preheat the oven to 350°F (175°C).
- Stuff apples with almond butter and sprinkle with cinnamon.
- Bake for 20 minutes until tender.

Prep time: 5 minutes

Cook time: 20 minutes

Nutritional Information:

- Calories: 150
- Protein: 2g
- Carbs: 25g
- Fats: 9g

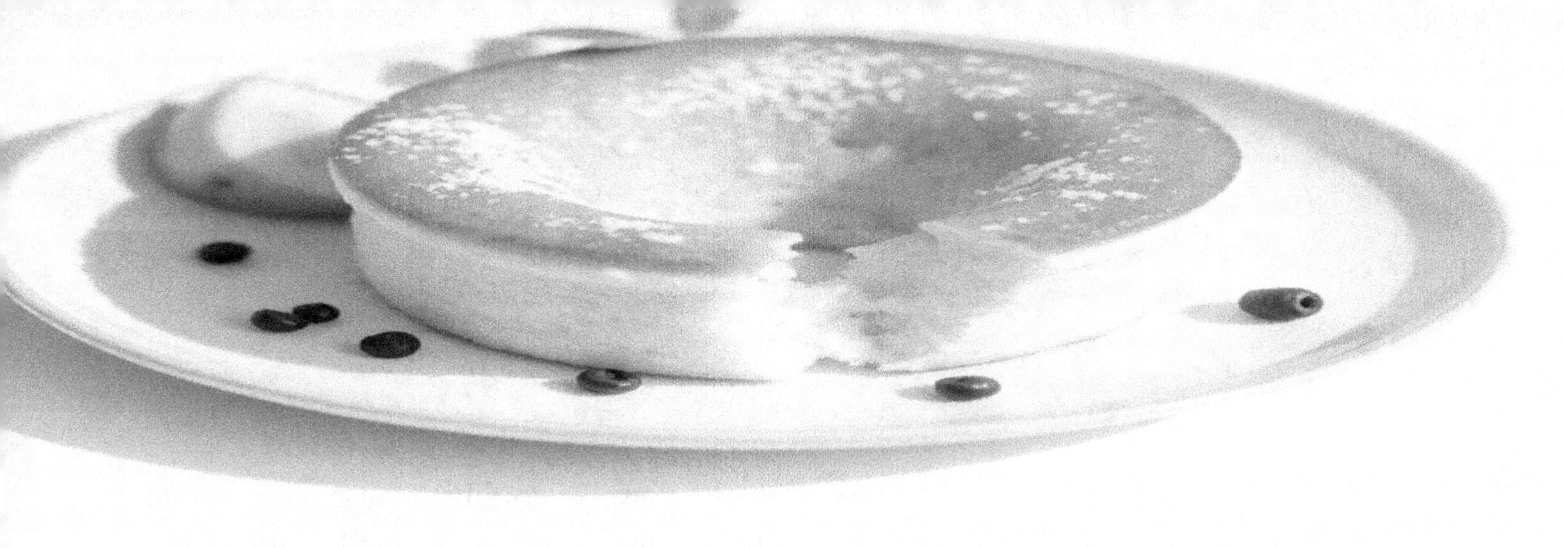

Coconut Flour Mug Cake

INGREDIENTS:

- 2 tbsp coconut flour
- 1 egg
- 1 tbsp honey
- 2 tbsp almond milk

INSTRUCTIONS:

- Mix all ingredients in a microwave-safe mug.
- Microwave on high for 1-2 minutes.
- Let cool slightly before serving.

Prep time: 3 minutes

Cook time: 2 minutes

Nutritional Information:

Calories: 180

Protein: 6g

Carbs: 12g

Fats: 14g

CHAPTER 12

Balancing on the Go

Life can get unpredictable—between work, family commitments, and social events, it's easy to feel like there's no time to focus on eating well. Add in the challenge of maintaining a healthy cortisol level while juggling a busy schedule, and it might seem like an impossible task. But with the right approach, you can balance everything without sacrificing your well-being.

In this chapter, we'll discuss simple strategies for managing your cortisol levels even when life throws curveballs. Whether you're traveling, dining out, or simply running between meetings, I'll share practical tips for eating on the go, offering you solutions that will make staying on track both easy and enjoyable.

The Common Challenges of Eating Out or Traveling

Eating out or traveling often brings its own set of challenges. With unpredictable menus, portion sizes, and the temptation to indulge in high-sugar or high-carb comfort foods, it's no wonder people struggle to maintain their healthy eating habits. For those working to keep their cortisol levels steady, these challenges can be even more pronounced. Cortisol, the stress hormone, spikes when you're in stressful situations—like rushing through an airport or trying to make a good impression at a work lunch. This means that choosing foods that stabilize blood sugar and reduce stress is even more important when you're away from home.

Here are a few common challenges people face when eating out or traveling:

- **Limited healthy options**: Many restaurants and fast food chains offer high-sugar, processed options that can spike blood sugar and lead to cortisol imbalances.
- **Large portion sizes**: Sometimes, the meals served at restaurants are far bigger than what you actually need, making it hard to control your calorie intake.
- **Temptation to indulge**: Social situations, especially meals with friends or family, can often lead to overindulgence or eating foods that aren't in line with your goals.

- **Unpredictable schedules**: Traveling often comes with tight timelines and little flexibility, making it tough to find time to eat the right foods.

Staying on Track in Unpredictable Situations

The good news is that even in the most chaotic situations, you can still make food choices that help keep your cortisol in check. A little planning and preparation can go a long way in helping you stay on track.

1. Plan Ahead with Portable Snacks

When you're on the go, the last thing you want is to be caught hungry without anything healthy to eat. Whether you're heading out for a day of errands or on a cross-country flight, packing snacks in advance is a smart strategy for maintaining balanced cortisol levels. The right portable snacks can stabilize blood sugar, avoid energy crashes, and keep you feeling satisfied for hours.

Here are some cortisol-friendly portable snacks to keep with you:

- **Nuts and Seeds**: These are rich in healthy fats and protein, which help keep blood sugar stable. A small handful of almonds, walnuts, or pumpkin seeds makes for an easy snack that won't spike your cortisol.
- **Hard-Boiled Eggs**: They're easy to prepare and pack, and they provide a great source of protein to keep you full and energized.
- **Protein Bars**: Look for bars with minimal sugar and high protein content. These can be a lifesaver when you need something quick and filling.
- **Veggie Chips or Fresh Veggies**: If you're craving something crunchy, grab some veggie chips (check the label to ensure there are no added sugars) or fresh veggies like carrots, celery, or cucumber.
- **Greek Yogurt with Berries**: Pack a small container of unsweetened Greek yogurt and add a handful of fresh berries. This provides protein, healthy fats, and antioxidants, helping to keep your stress levels in check.
- **Homemade Trail Mix**: Combine nuts, seeds, and a few pieces of dark chocolate or dried fruit for a balanced snack that provides fiber, fat, and protein.
- **Avocado and Crackers**: You can slice up an avocado and pair it with whole-grain crackers for a snack that's rich in healthy fats and fiber.

2. Easy-to-Order Meals at Restaurants

Dining out doesn't have to derail your healthy eating habits. Many restaurants offer healthier options, but it's important to know what to look for. You don't have to deprive yourself of dining out; you just need to make smart choices that will keep you on track with your goals.

Here are some tips for managing meals in social settings or at restaurants:

- **Look for Lean Proteins**: Most restaurants offer grilled chicken, fish, or other lean protein options. These meals are not only good for stabilizing blood sugar, but they also provide the essential nutrients your body needs to manage cortisol effectively.
- **Request Dressings on the Side**: Many dressings can be high in sugar or unhealthy fats. Asking for your dressing on the side gives you more control over how much you use.
- **Choose Roasted or Grilled Instead of Fried**: Fried foods are not only high in unhealthy fats, but they also cause a quick blood sugar spike, which can trigger cortisol spikes. Opt for roasted, grilled, or baked options instead.
- **Ask for Substitutions**: Don't hesitate to ask for a substitution if a dish comes with something you want to avoid (like fries or white bread). Ask for extra veggies, a side salad, or a baked potato instead. Most restaurants are happy to accommodate such requests.
- **Go for Whole Grains**: If your meal comes with rice, pasta, or bread, ask if they offer a whole-grain version. Whole grains, like brown rice or quinoa, are a better choice for stabilizing blood sugar compared to refined grains.
- **Be Mindful of Sauces and Sweets**: Sauces can often be high in sugar, so request them on the side if possible. Similarly, if you're tempted by dessert, consider sharing with a friend or opting for a small fruit bowl to satisfy your sweet tooth without overindulging.

Here are some meal ideas you can order when eating out:

- **Grilled Chicken Salad**: A grilled chicken salad with a variety of veggies and a light vinaigrette is a great go-to choice. It's loaded with fiber, protein, and healthy fats—helping to keep your cortisol steady.

- **Grilled Fish or Steak with Veggies**: Order a grilled piece of fish (like salmon) or lean steak, paired with steamed or roasted vegetables. This meal provides healthy fats, protein, and fiber.
- **Vegetable Stir-Fry with Tofu or Chicken**: Many Asian restaurants offer vegetable stir-fries. Choose one with lean protein and request it to be cooked in a small amount of healthy oil (like sesame or olive oil) to keep it light and healthy.
- **Egg-white Omelet with Veggies**: Breakfast isn't just for the morning! Most breakfast places offer egg-white omelets that you can load up with vegetables like spinach, mushrooms, and tomatoes.

3. Maintaining Balance in Social Situations

When you're out with friends or at a family gathering, there's often the temptation to indulge in foods that aren't the best for managing your cortisol levels. But it's possible to stay social without sacrificing your health goals.

Here are some strategies for managing social settings while keeping your cortisol in check:

- **Eat a Balanced Snack Before Going Out**: If you're heading to a dinner party or social gathering, eat a small, balanced snack beforehand. This will help you avoid arriving hungry and reaching for the unhealthy snacks that might be available.
- **Drink Water First**: Drink water before reaching for sugary drinks or alcoholic beverages. Staying hydrated helps prevent dehydration, which can lead to an increase in cortisol levels.
- **Share Plates**: If you're at a restaurant with friends and there are tempting dishes on the menu, suggest sharing. This way, you can enjoy the flavors without overeating.
- **Mind Your Alcohol**: While it's okay to enjoy an occasional glass of wine, remember that alcohol can increase cortisol levels. Stick to moderate consumption, and always drink plenty of water alongside it.
- **Be Mindful of Portions**: It's easy to get carried away when you're enjoying a meal with others. One way to manage this is to check in with yourself before ordering. Are you really hungry, or are you simply eating because food is available? It's okay to pass on the extras or to take home leftovers for later.

Eating on the go doesn't have to lead to a cortisol spike. By planning ahead with portable snacks and choosing the right options when dining out, you can maintain a balanced, healthy diet no matter how hectic life gets. Remember, small, sustainable changes can make a big impact. You can still enjoy life's social moments and eat well—it's all about making choices that work for you and your health goals. With these tips, you'll be well on your way to managing your cortisol and staying on track, no matter where life takes you.

4o mini

Part 5: Life After the Detox – Sustaining Your Hormonal Balance

CHAPTER 13

Beyond the Diet

So, you've made it through your detox, and now you're looking ahead. How do you keep the momentum going and maintain healthy cortisol levels in the long term? It's one thing to follow a plan for a few weeks or even a few months, but when it comes to creating lasting change, the key is consistency and adaptability.

In this chapter, we're going to talk about how you can continue to live a lifestyle that supports your cortisol health long after the initial detox phase. We'll explore how to adapt the principles of this detox into different stages of life and varying health goals. Whether you're dealing with a stressful job, navigating a busy family life, or working on a specific health target, you can make lasting changes that support your body's needs.

Building a Long-Term Lifestyle: It's About Consistency

While quick fixes can work in the short term, lasting change comes from consistent, sustainable habits. Adapting the principles you've learned during the detox phase into your everyday life will ensure that your cortisol levels remain balanced long-term.

One of the first things to recognize is that maintaining cortisol balance is not a one-size-fits-all approach. Each stage of life presents different challenges, and your body's needs will evolve over time. The good news is that the principles of this detox can be adapted to fit into whatever phase you're in.

Here's how you can build a lifestyle that supports your cortisol levels in the long run:

1. Prioritize Balanced Nutrition

It's easy to fall into unhealthy eating patterns once you're no longer following a strict detox, but keeping your cortisol levels balanced relies heavily on maintaining a nutrient-rich diet. You don't have to follow a strict detox plan forever, but you should continue to focus on whole, unprocessed foods that are rich in nutrients.

The idea is to make these foods a staple in your daily life:

- **Protein-Rich Foods**: Protein plays a critical role in balancing blood sugar and cortisol. Aim for high-quality protein sources, such as lean meats, fish, eggs, legumes, and plant-based options like tofu and tempeh. Protein helps to stabilize your blood sugar and keep your energy levels even, preventing the cortisol spikes that come with blood sugar crashes.
- **Healthy Fats**: Incorporate healthy fats into your diet, such as avocado, nuts, seeds, and olive oil. These fats help your body absorb essential nutrients and maintain steady hormone production, including cortisol. Healthy fats also provide long-lasting energy, which can help you get through your day without reaching for sugary snacks.
- **Complex Carbs**: Opt for whole grains, vegetables, and legumes. These foods are high in fiber, which helps slow the absorption of sugar into the bloodstream, preventing insulin spikes that trigger cortisol surges.

While it's important to maintain these basics, don't be afraid to indulge once in a while. It's about balance, not perfection.

2. Stay Active (But Don't Overdo It)

Exercise is an essential part of a healthy lifestyle, but when it comes to cortisol management, balance is key. While high-intensity workouts like running or weightlifting can be great for building strength and endurance, they can also increase cortisol levels if done excessively. Long periods of intense exercise can trigger the release of cortisol as a stress response.

However, the right amount of gentle movement can help to reduce cortisol and improve your overall well-being. Here are some tips for maintaining a healthy exercise routine:

- **Incorporate Low-Intensity Movement**: Gentle movement like walking, swimming, yoga, or light cycling can help to maintain a balanced cortisol level. These activities are great for relieving stress without overstimulating your body. The goal is to stay active and move your body every day, but without pushing it too hard.
- **Listen to Your Body**: Pay attention to how your body feels after exercise. If you're feeling more stressed or exhausted than usual, it may be a sign that you need to dial back the intensity. Aim for a routine that feels sustainable and energizing, rather than draining.

- **Prioritize Recovery**: Recovery is just as important as exercise itself. Adequate rest allows your cortisol levels to return to baseline and prevents burnout. Ensure you're getting enough sleep, stretching, and managing stress in between workouts to support your long-term health.

3. Manage Stress with Mindfulness and Relaxation

The key to keeping your cortisol levels steady over time is being proactive about stress management. Life will always throw curveballs, and stressors are inevitable. However, it's your response to stress that determines how it affects your health.

- **Practice Mindfulness**: Mindfulness and meditation have been shown to reduce cortisol levels significantly. These practices help you stay present, reduce overthinking, and create a sense of calm even in the midst of chaos. You don't have to spend hours meditating—start with just a few minutes each day. Whether it's a guided meditation, breathing exercises, or simply focusing on your breath, these techniques can work wonders for stress reduction.
- **Prioritize Rest**: Sleep is one of the most powerful tools you have to manage cortisol levels. Aim for 7-9 hours of quality sleep per night. Establish a bedtime routine that helps signal to your body that it's time to wind down. Avoid stimulants like caffeine in the evening, and create a calm, dark environment to promote better rest.
- **Take Breaks During the Day**: In today's fast-paced world, we often forget to take breaks. However, regular breaks are crucial for mental clarity and reducing cortisol. Whether it's stepping away from your desk for a few minutes or practicing deep breathing during a stressful meeting, taking a moment to reset can make a big difference.

4. Adapt the Plan to Different Life Stages and Health Goals

As you move through different stages of life, your cortisol management plan will need to evolve. Whether you're in your 30s and juggling career goals, in your 40s and managing family life, or in your 50s and focusing on longevity, understanding how to adjust your approach will help you maintain balance throughout life.

Here's how you can adapt the principles to your life:

- **In Your 30s**: During your 30s, you may be juggling work, family, and other responsibilities. It's easy for stress to build up, especially when balancing multiple commitments. During this stage, it's crucial to focus on building sustainable routines that support your health. Meal prepping, organizing your day, and staying consistent with movement will help you manage stress without feeling overwhelmed.

- **In Your 40s**: As you enter your 40s, your body's nutritional and hormonal needs may shift. Managing cortisol during this phase often requires a more mindful approach to nutrition, exercise, and rest. Focus on eating anti-inflammatory foods, managing stress, and incorporating restorative practices like yoga or Tai Chi to maintain energy levels and balance cortisol.
- **In Your 50s and Beyond**: In this stage, maintaining a steady cortisol level is important for healthy aging. As your metabolism naturally slows, you may need to adjust your diet and exercise routine to ensure you're not overstressing your body. Focus on maintaining muscle mass with strength training and continue to prioritize rest and relaxation to reduce the impact of stress on your body.

5. Encouraging Examples of Long-Term Success

It's important to remember that maintaining a balanced lifestyle is a journey, not a destination. Many people have successfully integrated these principles into their lives, leading to lasting improvements in their health, energy, and overall well-being. Here are a few examples:

- **Sarah, a Busy Mom**: Sarah, a working mother of two, initially struggled to find time for herself. After committing to small, daily habits like meal prepping and practicing mindfulness, she found herself feeling more energetic and less stressed. Over time, she noticed that her cortisol levels remained balanced, even on the busiest days.
- **Mark, a Corporate Executive**: Mark, a high-powered corporate executive, used to rely on caffeine to get through long workdays. After adopting a balanced diet and focusing on stress-reducing practices like deep breathing and yoga, he noticed that his energy improved and his stress levels decreased, even in high-pressure situations.
- **Emily, a Retiree**: Emily, now in her 60s, realized that her health needed a shift as she entered retirement. She focused on eating anti-inflammatory foods and committing to regular walks. The result? She found more peace in her day-to-day life, and her energy levels and mood stabilized as her cortisol levels balanced.

Maintaining healthy cortisol levels is an ongoing process, but with the right mindset, tools, and support, you can make it a part of your everyday life. By focusing on balanced nutrition, staying active, managing stress, and adapting the principles to fit different stages of life, you can ensure that you stay on track for long-term health and wellness. Remember, the goal isn't perfection; it's progress. Keep listening to your body, adjusting when needed, and celebrating your successes along the way. The journey to a balanced life is worth it, and it's yours to create.

CHAPTER 14

Your New Normal

How Reduced Stress and Balanced Hormones Translate into Lasting Energy, Better Health, and Weight Management

The day has finally come. You've worked through the changes, incorporated new habits into your life, and now, you're beginning to feel the results. Your stress levels have decreased, your energy is more consistent, and your hormones are starting to find balance. You might have started this journey for a specific goal, like weight loss or health improvements, but as you settle into this new lifestyle, you'll find that the benefits are much more far-reaching.

In this chapter, we're going to explore how reducing stress and balancing hormones can lead to lasting energy, better overall health, and a more sustainable approach to weight management. We'll also provide you with the tools, tips, and encouragement you need to embrace this way of living as a long-term investment in your well-being. The transformation you've started is not just a short-term fix—it's a new normal, and it's here to stay.

Embracing the New Routine

Adjusting to any new routine takes time, but the changes you've made are well worth the effort. You may have started by following a detox, altering your diet, or making small shifts to how you handle stress, but now that you've experienced the benefits of these adjustments, it's time to make them permanent. The key to this long-term success lies in embracing your new normal and reinforcing those positive habits.

Here are some tips to help you continue integrating your new routine into your daily life:

1. **Celebrate Small Wins**

   As you transition into your new lifestyle, celebrate the small victories. Maybe you're no longer feeling the mid-afternoon slump, or you're noticing that you're not reaching for sugary snacks the moment you feel stressed.

These wins, no matter how small, are steps in the right direction. Recognizing them will help you stay motivated as you continue to embrace your new habits.

2. **Create a Routine that Works for You**

   One of the easiest ways to maintain consistency is by creating a routine that fits your life. This doesn't mean rigidly scheduling every moment of your day, but rather setting up systems that make your healthy habits easier to maintain. Whether it's a quick morning meditation, a balanced breakfast, or a mid-afternoon walk, find simple habits that work for you and stick with them.

3. **Make Self-Care a Priority**

   Self-care isn't selfish; it's essential. Consistently prioritizing yourself—through sleep, mindfulness, exercise, and nutritious meals—will help you maintain the energy you need to thrive. When you take care of your mental, emotional, and physical health, you can give more to your family, your job, and every other part of your life.

4. **Plan Ahead for Success**

   As with any healthy habit, planning ahead is key. If you know you have a busy week ahead, try meal prepping or organizing your snacks. If you have social events coming up, plan your meals or review the menu ahead of time to make sure you can stay on track. By planning, you can ensure your new normal becomes second nature.

Now, let's talk about the incredible benefits that balanced hormones can bring to your life, beyond just weight management. Hormones are the messengers in your body, telling every system what to do, when to do it, and how to respond. When cortisol (your stress hormone) and other hormones like insulin, leptin, and ghrelin are in balance, your body functions more efficiently, making everything from weight loss to sleep improvements a whole lot easier.

1. **Steady Energy**

   Balanced hormones help maintain steady energy levels throughout the day. When your cortisol levels are balanced, you're less likely to experience those drastic energy crashes that come with high-stress moments. Instead, your energy is steady, which helps you feel more alert and focused without reaching for caffeine or sugary snacks. This means you can power through your day with a clearer mind and a body that's ready for whatever comes next.

2. **Improved Sleep**
   When your cortisol levels drop to a healthy range, your body can get into a more natural rhythm with your sleep-wake cycle. Good sleep is one of the most powerful tools you have for balancing hormones. With better sleep quality, you're not only helping regulate cortisol but also boosting other important hormones, like growth hormone and melatonin. As a result, you'll wake up feeling more refreshed, with a clearer mind and better overall mood.

3. **Better Digestion and Gut Health**
   Chronic stress wreaks havoc on the gut, leading to issues like bloating, discomfort, and even gut dysbiosis (an imbalance of gut bacteria). By keeping cortisol in check, you're allowing your digestive system to function more effectively. Your gut will have an easier time absorbing nutrients, and you'll likely feel less bloated and more comfortable after meals.

4. **Hormonal Balance for a Healthy Weight**
   One of the primary reasons people seek out a cortisol detox is weight management. Elevated cortisol levels, especially over the long term, can lead to increased fat storage, particularly around the abdomen. When your hormones are balanced, your body is better able to burn fat for energy, leading to more effective weight management. This isn't just about shedding pounds—it's about supporting your body's natural processes to achieve a healthy weight that's sustainable for the long term.

How Reduced Stress Enhances Health and Weight Management

Stress is one of the primary triggers of hormonal imbalance, particularly cortisol. When stress becomes chronic, it can affect nearly every aspect of your health. However, by effectively reducing stress and keeping cortisol levels steady, you can begin to notice improvements across the board:

1. **Mental Clarity**

   When your cortisol is under control, your mind feels clearer. You're less distracted by worries and more focused on the tasks at hand. This mental clarity helps you stay motivated to maintain your new habits, like meal prepping, exercising, or practicing mindfulness. Instead of feeling overwhelmed by life's demands, you'll approach each day with a calm, collected mindset.

2. **Improved Immune Function**

   Chronic stress weakens the immune system, making you more susceptible to illnesses. With lower cortisol levels and reduced stress, your immune system functions more optimally. This means fewer sick days and a stronger ability to fight off infections, allowing you to stay on track with your healthy habits.

3. **Sustained Motivation**

   As you see the improvements in your health, weight management, and overall well-being, your motivation will naturally rise. The benefits of stress reduction and hormone balancing will serve as ongoing reminders of why you started this journey in the first place. This sense of accomplishment and the positive feedback from your body will keep you moving forward.

4. **Emotional Resilience**

   Stress affects emotional well-being, leading to anxiety, irritability, and mood swings. By reducing stress and balancing hormones, you create emotional resilience. You'll feel more equipped to handle life's ups and downs without resorting to unhealthy coping mechanisms like overeating, over-exercising, or giving in to negative thoughts.

The Vision for the Future: A Long-Term Investment in Your Health

By now, you may be starting to feel the full impact of your new lifestyle. You've put in the effort, made the changes, and seen the results. Now, it's time to shift your mindset from short-term fixes to a long-term approach. This isn't just a phase or a detox that ends in a few weeks. It's a new chapter in your life, one that's built on sustainable habits and a focus on your overall well-being.

Imagine a future where you wake up feeling energized, balanced, and ready to tackle your day. Picture yourself confidently attending social events, knowing how to make smart food choices without feeling restricted. Visualize your body responding to your efforts, with your weight remaining steady and your energy never wavering. This is the life you're building—a life where stress no longer controls you, where hormones are balanced, and where your health is thriving.

The journey you're on is about much more than just weight loss or feeling better in the moment. It's about creating a lifestyle that you can maintain for years to come, one where your body, mind, and spirit are in harmony. When you embrace this new normal, you're investing in a healthier, happier future.

Encouraging Long-Term Success

Long-term success doesn't happen overnight. It's the result of consistent effort, self-compassion, and an ongoing commitment to maintaining the lifestyle changes you've made. There will be challenges along the way, but the tools and strategies you've learned will help you stay grounded and on track.

Remember that every day is a new opportunity to choose health and balance. Embrace the process, trust the journey, and celebrate the fact that you've already taken the most important step. Your new normal isn't just possible—it's here, and it's yours to enjoy for the rest of your life.

Conclusion

Your Journey to Lasting Health and Balance

As you reach the end of this book, it's important to take a moment and reflect on everything you've learned. What began as a journey to balance cortisol and achieve better health has turned into a roadmap for long-term wellness, energy, and well-being. This is not the end of your story—it's just the beginning.

Along the way, you've embraced changes that may have felt overwhelming at first but now feel like second nature. From understanding the science behind cortisol and its impact on your health, to implementing a meal plan that supports your body's natural rhythms, to finding balance in a busy life, you've already made incredible strides. But here's the truth: this isn't a quick fix, and it isn't about perfection. It's about progress.

The tools, recipes, and strategies shared in these pages are not temporary fixes. They're meant to be woven into the fabric of your life as you continue to grow, learn, and adjust. Health is not a destination—it's a lifelong journey. And with the foundation you've laid, you're now equipped to create a balanced, healthy, and empowered life.

Remember, the key to success is consistency, not perfection. There will be moments when life feels chaotic, when stress creeps back in, or when you feel tempted to fall into old habits. But those moments don't define you—they're just part of the journey. You now have the tools to reset, to recalibrate, and to continue moving forward with a clear sense of purpose.

Take pride in the small victories along the way. The quiet moments of feeling energized in the morning, the satisfaction of choosing a nourishing meal instead of a quick fix, the joy of a calmer mind despite the busyness of life—these are the markers of lasting change. And they will keep coming, day after day, as you continue to nurture yourself and make choices that support your health.

You've invested in yourself, in your health, and in your future. The habits you've created will continue to support you, helping you thrive in every area of your life. The balance you've worked so hard to achieve will become the new normal—a place where you feel grounded, vibrant, and empowered.

So, take a deep breath, acknowledge how far you've come, and trust that this journey has already made a lasting impact. You have everything you need to continue living a life full of energy, vitality, and balance. The tools and habits you've adopted will continue to serve you as you evolve, helping you stay steady and resilient, no matter what life throws your way.

Your journey to lasting health isn't a destination; it's a way of living. Keep embracing it, one day at a time, and know that you're building a foundation for a lifetime of wellness.

The best is yet to come. Keep moving forward with confidence, knowing you have the power to create the vibrant life you deserve.

MY SPECIAL GIFT TO YOU, THANK YOU! FOR CHOOSING THIS BOOK

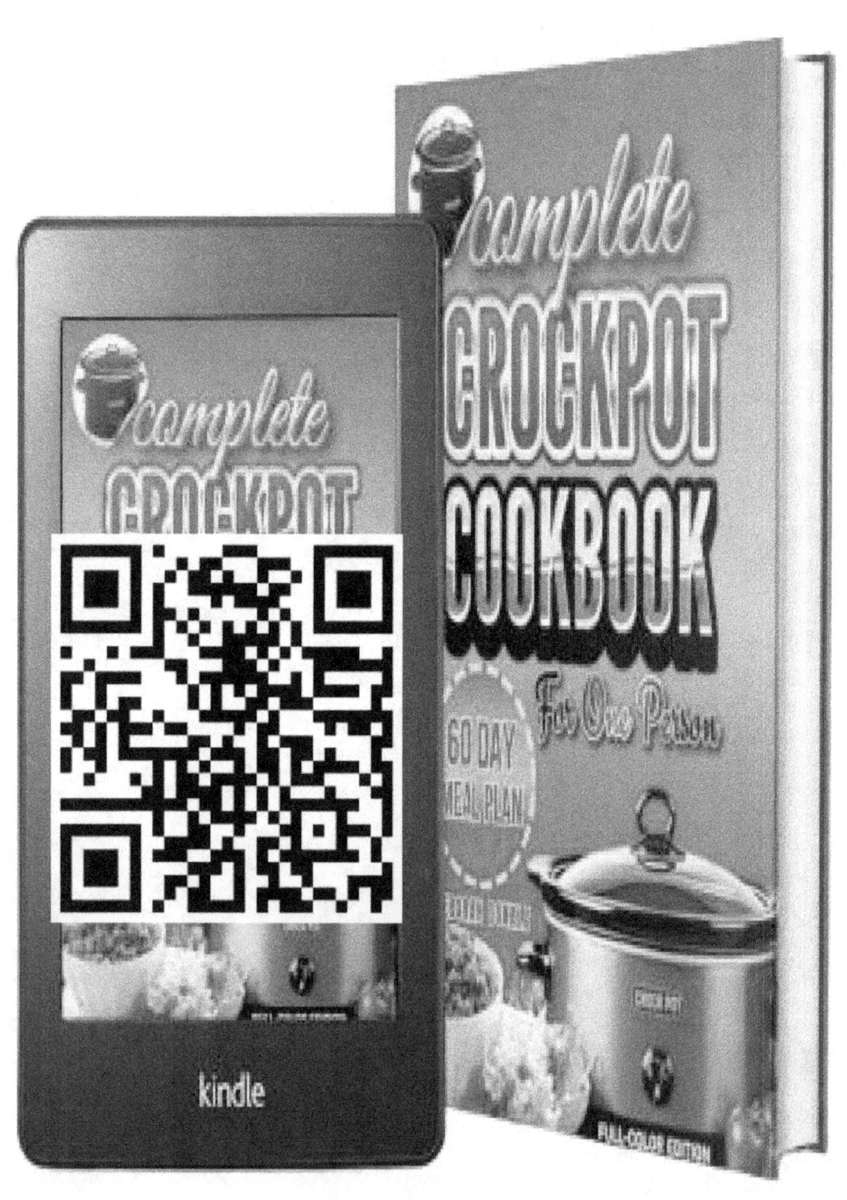

MONDAY

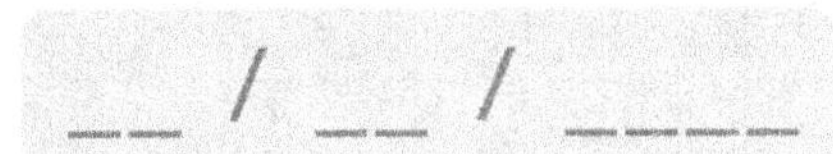

TRACK TODAY		
	BEFORE	AFTER
BREAK FAST		
LUNCH		
SNACK		
DINNER		

NOTE

MOOD:

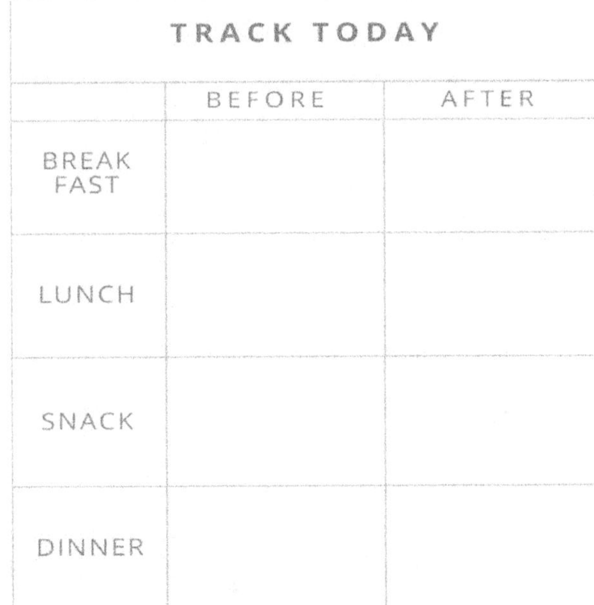

TUESDAY

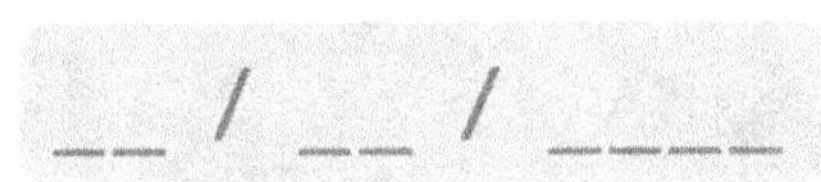

TRACK TODAY		
	BEFORE	AFTER
BREAK FAST		
LUNCH		
SNACK		
DINNER		

NOTE

MOOD:

WEDNESDAY

__ / __ / ____

TRACK TODAY	BEFORE	AFTER
BREAK FAST		
LUNCH		
SNACK		
DINNER		

NOTE:

MOOD:

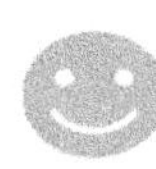 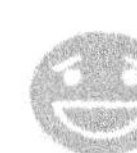   

THURSDAY

__ / __ / ____

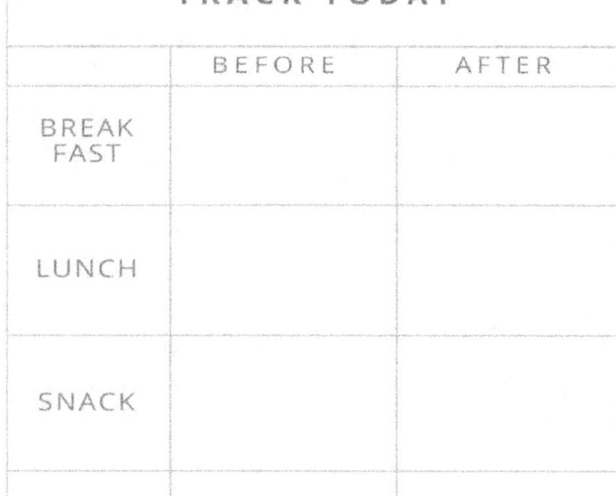

TRACK TODAY	BEFORE	AFTER
BREAK FAST		
LUNCH		
SNACK		
DINNER		

NOTE:

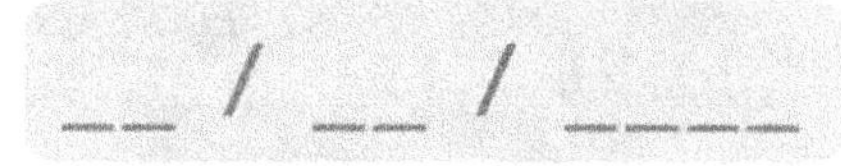

MOOD:

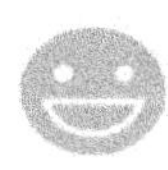  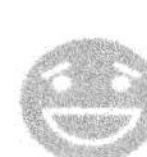   

FRIDAY

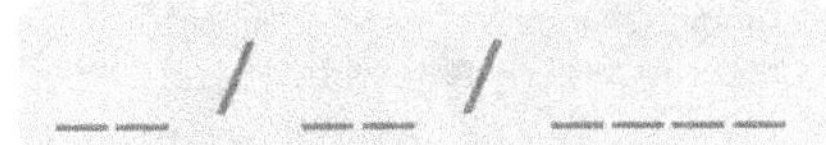

<table>
<tr><th colspan="3">TRACK TODAY</th></tr>
<tr><td></td><td>BEFORE</td><td>AFTER</td></tr>
<tr><td>BREAK FAST</td><td></td><td></td></tr>
<tr><td>LUNCH</td><td></td><td></td></tr>
<tr><td>SNACK</td><td></td><td></td></tr>
<tr><td>DINNER</td><td></td><td></td></tr>
</table>

__ / __ / ____

NOTE:

MOOD:

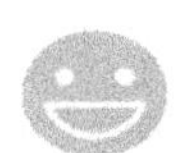  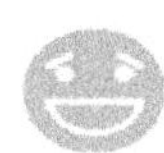  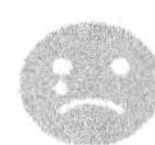 

SATURDAY

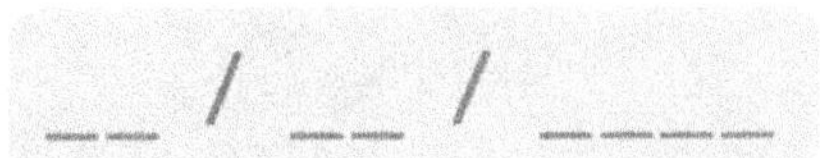

<table>
<tr><th colspan="3">TRACK TODAY</th></tr>
<tr><td></td><td>BEFORE</td><td>AFTER</td></tr>
<tr><td>BREAK FAST</td><td></td><td></td></tr>
<tr><td>LUNCH</td><td></td><td></td></tr>
<tr><td>SNACK</td><td></td><td></td></tr>
<tr><td>DINNER</td><td></td><td></td></tr>
</table>

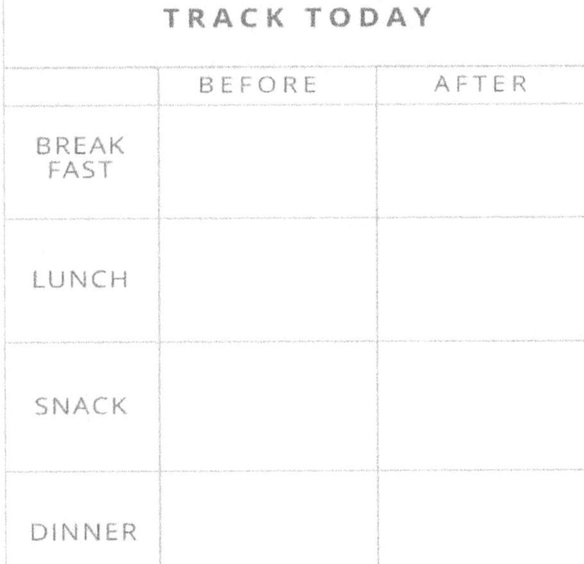

__ / __ / ____

NOTE:

MOOD:

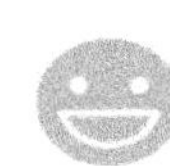  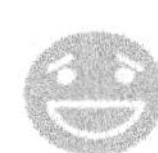   

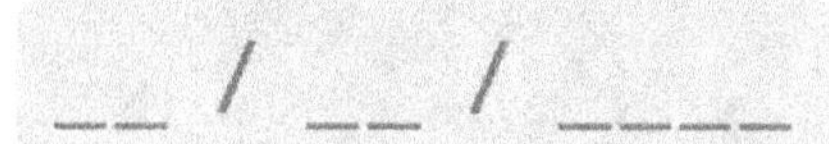

TRACK TODAY

	BEFORE	AFTER
BREAK FAST		
LUNCH		
SNACK		
DINNER		

NOTE:

MOOD:

WEEKLY SUMMARY

Weight Tracker

START	END

Weight Tracker

START	END

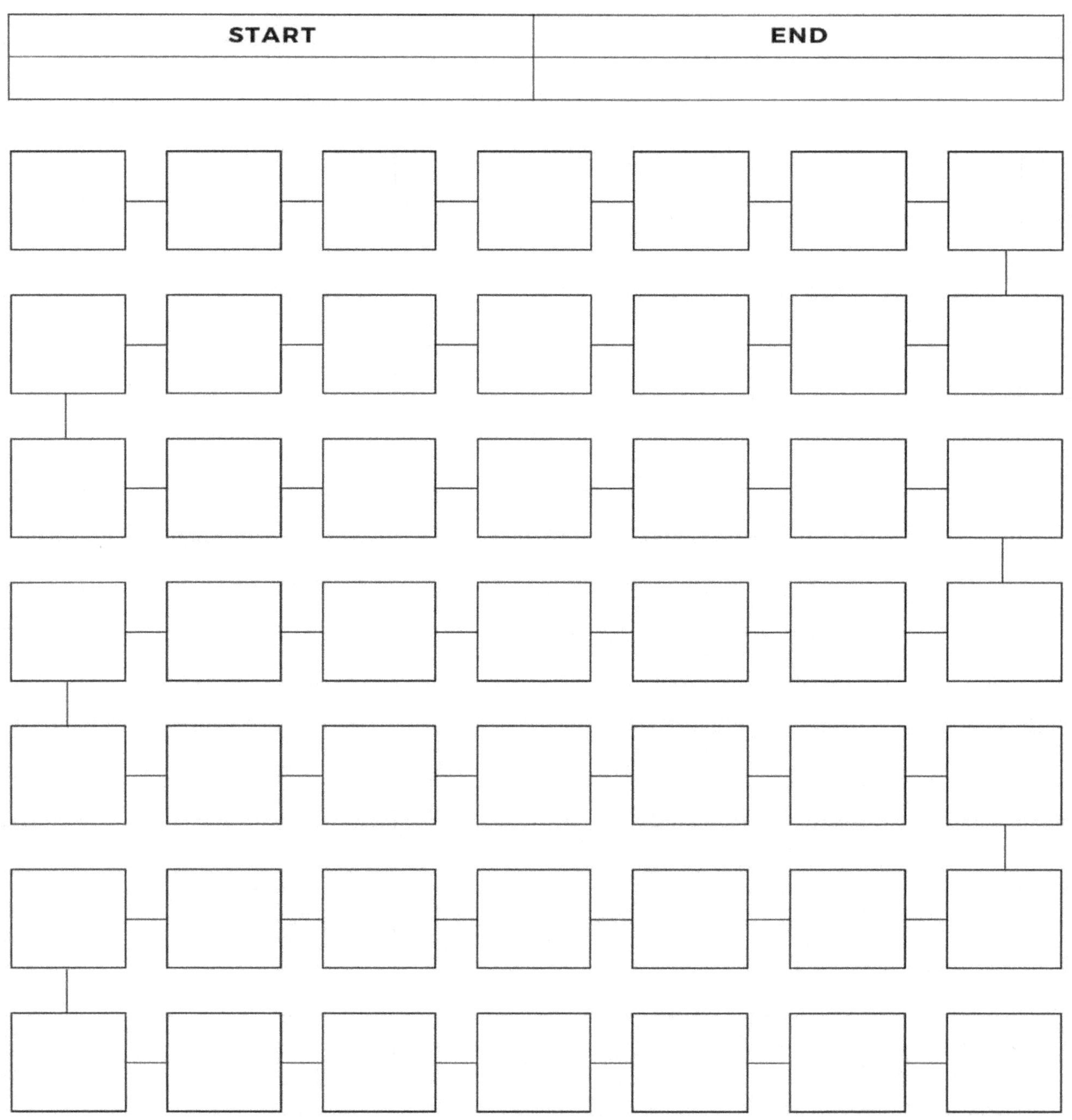

Weight Tracker

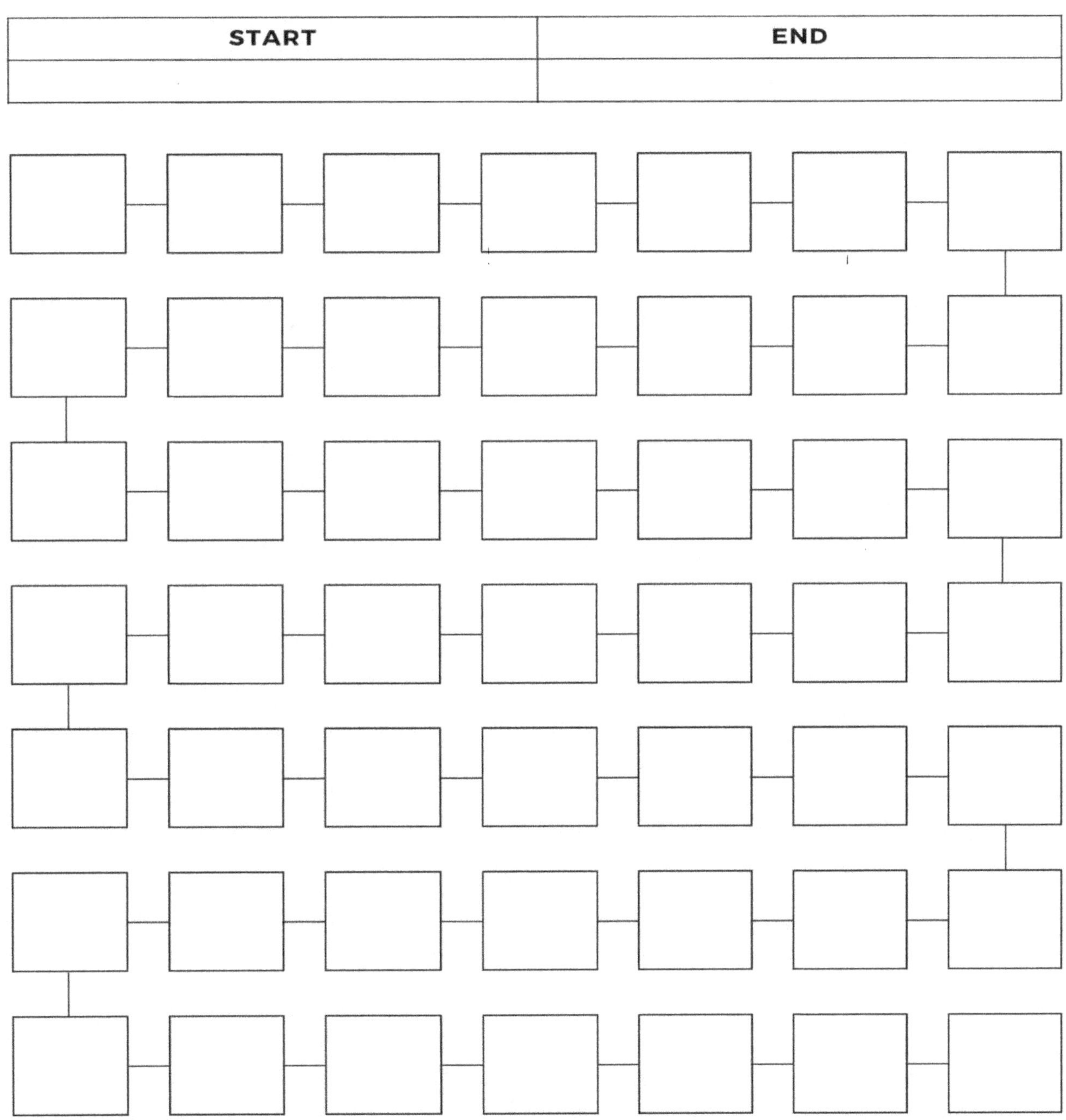